Introductions

Welcome to the **One-Pan Cookbook For Women**, where delicious meals meet convenience and health! This cookbook is designed with the modern woman in mind, offering a collection of 100 simple, fast, and nutritious recipes that can be prepared using just one pan. Whether you're a busy professional, a multitasking mom, or simply someone who loves good food without the hassle, this book is your ultimate kitchen companion.

In today's fast-paced world, finding the time to prepare wholesome meals can be a challenge. Yet, as women, we understand the importance of nourishing ourselves and our loved ones with balanced, homemade dishes. This cookbook is here to make that task easier than ever before. With just one pan, you can create mouthwatering meals that not only taste great but also support your health and well-being.

Gone are the days of juggling multiple pots and pans, spending hours in the kitchen, and dealing with a pile of dishes afterward. In this book, you'll discover a treasure trove of recipes that require minimal prep work, minimal cleanup, and maximum flavor. From hearty breakfasts and satisfying lunches to comforting dinners and indulgent desserts, there's something for every palate and every occasion.

But this cookbook is more than just a collection of recipes. It's a celebration of women's empowerment in the kitchen. It's about reclaiming our time, simplifying our lives, and embracing the joy of cooking without the stress. It's about finding balance in a world that often feels chaotic, one delicious meal at a time.

Whether you're a novice cook or a seasoned chef, you'll find plenty of inspiration within these pages to elevate your culinary repertoire. So grab your favorite pan, sharpen your knives, and let's embark on a culinary journey that's as delightful as it is effortless. Here's to good food, good health, and the power of women in the kitchen!

1. Chicken Stir-Fry with Vegetables

Ingredients:
- 1 tablespoon vegetable oil
- 1 pound boneless, skinless chicken breasts, thinly sliced
- Salt and pepper to taste
- 2 cloves garlic, minced
- 1 bell pepper, thinly sliced
- 1 small onion, thinly sliced
- 1 cup broccoli florets
- 1 cup sliced mushrooms
- 1/4 cup soy sauce
- 2 tablespoons oyster sauce (optional)
- 1 tablespoon sesame oil
- Cooked rice, for serving

Instructions:

1. Heat the vegetable oil in a large skillet over medium-high heat.

2. Season the chicken slices with salt and pepper, then add them to the skillet. Cook for 5-6 minutes, or until the chicken is browned and cooked through. Remove the chicken from the skillet and set it aside.

3. In the same skillet, add a little more oil if needed, then add the minced garlic, bell pepper, and onion. Cook for 2-3 minutes, stirring frequently, until the vegetables start to soften.

4. Add the broccoli florets and sliced mushrooms to the skillet. Cook for an additional 3-4 minutes, or until the vegetables are tender-crisp.

5. Return the cooked chicken to the skillet. Stir in the soy sauce and oyster sauce, if using. Cook for another 2-3 minutes, stirring occasionally, until everything is heated through and well combined.

6. Drizzle the sesame oil over the stir-fry and toss to coat.

7. Serve the chicken stir-fry with vegetables over cooked rice.

Enjoy your delicious and easy single-skillet chicken stir-fry!

2. Vegetable Fried Rice

Ingredients:

- 2 tablespoons vegetable oil
- 2 eggs, lightly beaten
- 2 cups cooked rice (preferably day-old)
- 1 cup mixed vegetables (such as peas, carrots, corn, and green beans), fresh or frozen
- 2 cloves garlic, minced
- 2 green onions, chopped
- 2 tablespoons soy sauce
- Salt and pepper to taste
- Optional: cooked chicken, shrimp, or tofu for added protein

Instructions:

1. Heat 1 tablespoon of vegetable oil in a large skillet over medium heat. Pour the beaten eggs into the skillet and cook, stirring gently, until they are scrambled. Remove the scrambled eggs from the skillet and set them aside.

2. In the same skillet, add the remaining tablespoon of vegetable oil. Add the minced garlic and chopped green onions, and cook for 1-2 minutes until fragrant.

3. Add the mixed vegetables to the skillet. If using frozen vegetables, you can add them directly from the freezer. Cook for 3-4 minutes, or until the vegetables are tender.

4. If you're adding cooked chicken, shrimp, or tofu, add it to the skillet at this point and cook until heated through.

5. Add the cooked rice to the skillet, breaking up any clumps with a spoon or spatula. Stir-fry the rice and vegetables together for 2-3 minutes, allowing the rice to heat through.

6. Pour the soy sauce over the rice and vegetables. Add salt and pepper to taste. Stir well to combine, making sure the soy sauce is evenly distributed.

7. Return the scrambled eggs to the skillet, breaking them up into smaller pieces as you stir them into the rice.

8. Cook for an additional 1-2 minutes, or until everything is heated through and well combined.

9. Taste and adjust seasoning if necessary.

10. Serve the vegetable fried rice hot, optionally garnished with additional chopped green onions.

3. Shakshuka with Feta Cheese

Ingredients:
- 2 tablespoons olive oil
- 1 onion, chopped
- 1 red bell pepper, chopped
- 2 cloves garlic, minced
- 1 teaspoon ground cumin
- 1 teaspoon paprika
- 1/2 teaspoon chili powder (adjust to taste)
- 1 can (14 ounces) diced tomatoes
- Salt and pepper to taste
- 4-6 large eggs
- 1/4 cup crumbled feta cheese
- Chopped fresh parsley or cilantro for garnish (optional)
- Crusty bread or pita bread, for serving

Instructions:

1. Heat the olive oil in a large skillet over medium heat. Add the chopped onion and red bell pepper. Cook for 5-7 minutes, stirring occasionally, until the vegetables are softened.

2. Add the minced garlic, ground cumin, paprika, and chili powder to the skillet. Cook for an additional 1-2 minutes, stirring constantly, until fragrant.

3. Pour the diced tomatoes (with their juices) into the skillet. Stir to combine with the vegetables and spices. Season with salt and pepper to taste.

4. Simmer the tomato mixture for 10-15 minutes, or until it has thickened slightly.

5. Using a spoon, create small wells in the tomato mixture for each egg. Crack an egg into each well.

6. Cover the skillet and cook for 5-7 minutes, or until the egg whites are set but the yolks are still runny (or to your desired doneness).

7. Sprinkle the crumbled feta cheese over the top of the shakshuka.

8. Garnish with chopped fresh parsley or cilantro, if desired.

9. Serve the shakshuka hot, straight from the skillet, with crusty bread or pita bread for dipping.

4. Spinach and Feta Frittata

Ingredients:
- 6 large eggs
- 1/4 cup milk or cream
- Salt and pepper to taste
- 1 tablespoon olive oil
- 2 cups fresh spinach leaves, roughly chopped
- 1/2 cup crumbled feta cheese
- 1/4 cup diced onion
- 2 cloves garlic, minced
- Optional: chopped fresh herbs such as parsley or dill

Instructions:

1. Preheat your oven broiler on high.

2. In a mixing bowl, whisk together the eggs, milk or cream, salt, and pepper until well combined. Set aside.

3. Heat the olive oil in a large oven-safe skillet over medium heat. Add the diced onion and minced garlic. Cook for 2-3 minutes, or until the onion is softened and fragrant.

4. Add the chopped spinach to the skillet. Cook for 1-2 minutes, stirring occasionally, until the spinach wilts.

5. Spread the spinach mixture evenly across the bottom of the skillet. Pour the egg mixture over the spinach.

6. Sprinkle the crumbled feta cheese evenly over the top of the egg mixture.

7. Cook the frittata on the stovetop for 3-4 minutes, or until the edges start to set.

8. Transfer the skillet to the preheated oven and broil for 3-5 minutes, or until the top is golden brown and the center is set. Keep a close eye on it to prevent burning.

9. Once the frittata is cooked to your liking, remove it from the oven and let it cool for a few minutes.

10. Optionally, garnish with chopped fresh herbs before serving.

11. Slice the frittata into wedges and serve warm or at room temperature.

5. Spaghetti Aglio e Olio

Ingredients:
- 8 ounces spaghetti
- 1/4 cup extra virgin olive oil
- 4 cloves garlic, thinly sliced
- 1/2 teaspoon red pepper flakes (adjust to taste)
- Salt to taste
- 1/4 cup chopped fresh parsley
- Grated Parmesan cheese for serving (optional)

Instructions:

1. Cook the spaghetti according to the package instructions until al dente. Reserve about 1/2 cup of the pasta cooking water, then drain the spaghetti and set it aside.

2. In the same skillet used to cook the spaghetti, heat the extra virgin olive oil over medium heat.

3. Add the thinly sliced garlic and red pepper flakes to the skillet. Cook for 1-2 minutes, stirring constantly, until the garlic is golden and fragrant. Be careful not to let the garlic burn.

4. Add the cooked spaghetti to the skillet, tossing it with the garlic and oil to coat evenly. If the spaghetti seems dry, add a splash of the reserved pasta cooking water to moisten it.

5. Season the spaghetti aglio e olio with salt to taste. Toss well to combine.

6. Remove the skillet from the heat and stir in the chopped fresh parsley.

7. Serve the spaghetti aglio e olio hot, optionally garnished with grated Parmesan cheese.

Enjoy your delicious and easy single-skillet spaghetti aglio e olio!

6. Creamy Tuscan Garlic Chicken

Ingredients:
- 4 boneless, skinless chicken breasts
- Salt and pepper to taste
- 2 tablespoons olive oil
- 4 cloves garlic, minced
- 1 cup cherry tomatoes, halved
- 1 cup spinach leaves
- 1 cup heavy cream
- 1/2 cup grated Parmesan cheese
- 1 teaspoon Italian seasoning
- Salt and pepper to taste
- Fresh chopped parsley for garnish (optional)

Instructions:

1. Season both sides of the chicken breasts with salt and pepper.

2. Heat olive oil in a large skillet over medium-high heat. Add the chicken breasts to the skillet and cook for about 6-7 minutes on each side, or until golden brown and cooked through. Remove the chicken from the skillet and set aside.

3. In the same skillet, add minced garlic and cook for about 1 minute until fragrant.

4. Add cherry tomatoes to the skillet and cook for another 2-3 minutes until they start to soften.

5. Stir in spinach leaves and cook until wilted.

6. Reduce the heat to medium-low. Pour in the heavy cream, grated Parmesan cheese, and Italian seasoning. Stir well until the sauce is creamy and well combined. Season with salt and pepper to taste.

7. Return the cooked chicken breasts to the skillet and spoon some of the creamy sauce over the chicken.

8. Allow the chicken to simmer in the sauce for another 2-3 minutes until heated through.

9. Garnish with fresh chopped parsley, if desired, before serving.

10. Serve the Creamy Tuscan Garlic Chicken hot, with your favorite side dishes like pasta, rice, or crusty bread.

7. Vegetarian Chili

Ingredients:

- 2 tablespoons olive oil
- 1 onion, diced
- 2 cloves garlic, minced
- 1 bell pepper, diced
- 1 zucchini, diced
- 1 carrot, diced
- 1 can (15 ounces) black beans, drained and rinsed
- 1 can (15 ounces) kidney beans, drained and rinsed
- 1 can (15 ounces) diced tomatoes
- 1 cup vegetable broth
- 2 tablespoons tomato paste
- 1 tablespoon chili powder
- 1 teaspoon ground cumin
- 1 teaspoon paprika
- Salt and pepper to taste
- Optional toppings: shredded cheese, chopped green onions, sour cream, avocado slices, cilantro, lime wedges

Instructions:

1. Heat the olive oil in a large skillet over medium heat.

2. Add the diced onion and minced garlic to the skillet. Cook for 2-3 minutes, or until the onion is softened and fragrant.

3. Add the diced bell pepper, zucchini, and carrot to the skillet. Cook for another 5 minutes, or until the vegetables are slightly tender.

4. Stir in the black beans, kidney beans, diced tomatoes, vegetable broth, tomato paste, chili powder, ground cumin, paprika, salt, and pepper.

5. Bring the chili to a simmer and let it cook for 15-20 minutes, stirring occasionally, until the vegetables are cooked through and the flavors are well combined. If the chili becomes too thick, you can add more vegetable broth as needed.

6. Taste and adjust seasoning if necessary.

7. Serve the vegetarian chili hot, topped with your favorite optional toppings such as shredded cheese, chopped green onions, sour cream, avocado slices, cilantro, and lime wedges.

8. One-Pan Lemon Herb Chicken and Asparagus

Ingredients:
- 4 boneless, skinless chicken breasts
- Salt and pepper to taste
- 2 tablespoons olive oil, divided
- 1 bunch asparagus, tough ends trimmed and cut into 2-inch pieces
- 4 cloves garlic, minced
- Zest and juice of 1 lemon
- 1 teaspoon dried thyme
- 1 teaspoon dried rosemary
- 1/2 cup chicken broth or white wine
- Optional: Fresh parsley for garnish

Instructions:

1. Season both sides of the chicken breasts with salt and pepper.

2. Heat 1 tablespoon of olive oil in a large skillet over medium-high heat. Add the chicken breasts to the skillet and cook for about 5-6 minutes on each side, or until golden brown and cooked through. Remove the chicken from the skillet and set aside.

3. In the same skillet, add the remaining tablespoon of olive oil. Add the minced garlic and cook for about 1 minute until fragrant.

4. Add the asparagus to the skillet and cook for about 3-4 minutes, stirring occasionally, until slightly tender.

5. Stir in the lemon zest, lemon juice, dried thyme, and dried rosemary.

6. Pour in the chicken broth or white wine and stir, scraping up any browned bits from the bottom of the skillet.

7. Return the cooked chicken breasts to the skillet, nestling them among the asparagus.

8. Cover the skillet and let everything simmer together for another 5 minutes, allowing the flavors to meld and the chicken to heat through.

9. Taste and adjust seasoning if necessary.

10. Serve the one-pan lemon herb chicken and asparagus hot, optionally garnished with fresh parsley.

Enjoy your delicious and easy single-skillet one-pan lemon herb chicken and asparagus!

9. Sweet Potato and Black Bean Skillet

Ingredients:

- 2 medium sweet potatoes, peeled and diced into cubes
- 1 tablespoon olive oil
- 1 small onion, diced
- 2 cloves garlic, minced
- 1 red bell pepper, diced
- 1 can (15 ounces) black beans, drained and rinsed
- 1 teaspoon ground cumin
- 1 teaspoon chili powder
- Salt and pepper to taste
- 1/2 cup vegetable broth or water
- Juice of 1 lime
- Optional toppings: chopped fresh cilantro, sliced avocado, sour cream, shredded cheese

Instructions:

1. Heat the olive oil in a large skillet over medium heat.

2. Add the diced sweet potatoes to the skillet. Cook for about 8-10 minutes, stirring occasionally, until the sweet potatoes are tender and slightly browned.

3. Add the diced onion, minced garlic, and diced red bell pepper to the skillet. Cook for another 3-4 minutes until the vegetables are softened and fragrant.

4. Stir in the drained and rinsed black beans, ground cumin, and chili powder. Season with salt and pepper to taste.

5. Pour in the vegetable broth or water, stirring to combine all the ingredients.

6. Cover the skillet and let the mixture simmer for about 5-7 minutes, or until the sweet potatoes are fully cooked and the flavors have melded together.

7. Squeeze the lime juice over the skillet and stir to combine.

8. Taste and adjust seasoning if necessary.

9. Serve the sweet potato and black bean skillet hot, optionally topped with chopped fresh cilantro, sliced avocado, sour cream, or shredded cheese.

Enjoy your delicious and easy single-skillet sweet potato and black bean skillet!

10. Mushroom and Spinach Quesadillas

Ingredients:
- 4 large flour tortillas
- 2 cups sliced mushrooms
- 2 cups fresh spinach leaves
- 1 cup shredded cheese (such as mozzarella, cheddar, or a Mexican blend)
- 1 tablespoon olive oil
- Salt and pepper to taste
- Optional toppings: salsa, sour cream, guacamole

Instructions:

1. Heat the olive oil in a large skillet over medium heat.

2. Add the sliced mushrooms to the skillet and cook for about 5-7 minutes, stirring occasionally, until they are tender and lightly browned. Season with salt and pepper to taste.

3. Add the fresh spinach leaves to the skillet and cook for another 1-2 minutes, or until the spinach is wilted. Remove the skillet from the heat and set aside.

4. Place a flour tortilla in the skillet over medium heat. Sprinkle some shredded cheese evenly over one half of the tortilla.

5. Spoon some of the cooked mushroom and spinach mixture over the cheese.

6. Sprinkle additional cheese over the mushroom and spinach mixture.

7. Fold the empty half of the tortilla over the filling to form a half-moon shape.

8. Cook the quesadilla for 2-3 minutes on each side, or until the tortilla is golden brown and the cheese is melted.

9. Remove the quesadilla from the skillet and transfer it to a cutting board. Let it cool for a minute or two, then slice it into wedges.

10. Repeat the process with the remaining tortillas and filling ingredients.

11. Serve the mushroom and spinach quesadillas hot, optionally topped with salsa, sour cream, or guacamole

11. Cajun Shrimp and Sausage Skillet

Ingredients:
- 1 pound large shrimp, peeled and deveined
- 8 ounces smoked sausage or andouille sausage, sliced
- 1 tablespoon Cajun seasoning
- 2 tablespoons olive oil
- 1 onion, diced
- 1 bell pepper, diced
- 2 cloves garlic, minced
- 1 can (14.5 ounces) diced tomatoes, drained
- 1 cup chicken broth
- Salt and pepper to taste
- Cooked rice, for serving
- Optional garnish: chopped green onions, chopped parsley

Instructions:

1. In a bowl, toss the shrimp with Cajun seasoning until evenly coated. Set aside.

2. Heat 1 tablespoon of olive oil in a large skillet over medium-high heat. Add the sliced sausage and cook until browned, about 3-4 minutes per side. Remove the sausage from the skillet and set aside.

3. In the same skillet, add the remaining tablespoon of olive oil. Add the diced onion and bell pepper. Cook for 3-4 minutes until softened.

4. Add the minced garlic to the skillet and cook for another 1-2 minutes until fragrant.

5. Add the diced tomatoes to the skillet and cook for 2-3 minutes.

6. Pour in the chicken broth and bring to a simmer.

7. Return the cooked sausage to the skillet and stir to combine with the vegetables.

8. Add the seasoned shrimp to the skillet in an even layer. Cook for 2-3 minutes per side until the shrimp are pink and cooked through.

9. Season with salt and pepper to taste.

10. Serve the Cajun shrimp and sausage skillet hot over cooked rice.

11. Garnish with chopped green onions and chopped parsley, if desired.

12. Caprese Chicken

Ingredients:
- 4 boneless, skinless chicken breasts
- Salt and pepper to taste
- 2 tablespoons olive oil
- 2 cloves garlic, minced
- 1 cup cherry tomatoes, halved
- 8 ounces fresh mozzarella cheese, sliced
- Balsamic glaze (store-bought or homemade)
- Fresh basil leaves, thinly sliced, for garnish

Instructions:

1. Season both sides of the chicken breasts with salt and pepper.

2. Heat olive oil in a large skillet over medium-high heat.

3. Add the seasoned chicken breasts to the skillet and cook for about 6-7 minutes on each side, or until they are golden brown and cooked through. Remove the chicken from the skillet and set aside.

4. In the same skillet, add minced garlic and cook for about 1 minute until fragrant.

5. Add cherry tomatoes to the skillet and cook for another 2-3 minutes until they start to soften.

6. Return the cooked chicken breasts to the skillet, arranging them in a single layer.

7. Top each chicken breast with a slice of fresh mozzarella cheese.

8. Cover the skillet and let it cook for 2-3 minutes, or until the cheese is melted and bubbly.

9. Drizzle balsamic glaze over the chicken breasts.

10. Garnish with thinly sliced fresh basil leaves.

11. Serve the Caprese Chicken hot, optionally with a side of cooked pasta or a salad.

Enjoy your delicious and easy single-skillet Caprese Chicken!

13. Garlic Butter Steak and Potatoes

Ingredients:

- 1 pound sirloin steak, cut into bite-sized pieces
- Salt and pepper to taste
- 2 tablespoons olive oil
- 3 tablespoons butter, divided
- 3 cloves garlic, minced
- 1 pound baby potatoes, halved or quartered
- 1 teaspoon dried thyme (or other herbs of your choice)
- Chopped fresh parsley for garnish (optional)

Instructions:

1. Season the steak pieces with salt and pepper to taste.

2. Heat olive oil in a large skillet over medium-high heat.

3. Add the seasoned steak pieces to the skillet and cook for about 2-3 minutes on each side, or until they are browned to your liking. Remove the steak from the skillet and set aside.

4. In the same skillet, add 1 tablespoon of butter and minced garlic. Cook for about 1 minute until the garlic is fragrant.

5. Add the halved baby potatoes to the skillet, arranging them in a single layer. Cook for about 8-10 minutes, stirring occasionally, until the potatoes are golden brown and tender.

6. Stir in the dried thyme and season with additional salt and pepper if needed.

7. Push the potatoes to one side of the skillet and return the cooked steak to the skillet, arranging it next to the potatoes.

8. Add the remaining 2 tablespoons of butter to the skillet, allowing it to melt and coat the steak and potatoes.

9. Cook for another 1-2 minutes, stirring gently, to coat the steak and potatoes with the garlic butter sauce.

10. Garnish with chopped fresh parsley, if desired.

11. Serve the Garlic Butter Steak and Potatoes hot, optionally with a side of steamed vegetables or a salad.

14. Pasta Primavera

Ingredients:

- 8 ounces pasta (such as spaghetti or fettuccine)
- 2 tablespoons olive oil
- 2 cloves garlic, minced
- 1 onion, thinly sliced
- 1 bell pepper, thinly sliced
- 1 zucchini, thinly sliced
- 1 yellow squash, thinly sliced
- 1 cup cherry tomatoes, halved
- Salt and pepper to taste
- 1/2 cup grated Parmesan cheese
- Fresh basil leaves, thinly sliced, for garnish

Instructions:

1. Cook the pasta according to the package instructions until al dente. Reserve about 1/2 cup of the pasta cooking water, then drain the pasta and set it aside.

2. In the same skillet used to cook the pasta, heat the olive oil over medium heat.

3. Add the minced garlic and thinly sliced onion to the skillet. Cook for 2-3 minutes until the onion is softened and fragrant.

4. Add the thinly sliced bell pepper, zucchini, and yellow squash to the skillet. Cook for another 5-7 minutes, stirring occasionally, until the vegetables are tender-crisp.

5. Stir in the halved cherry tomatoes and cook for an additional 2-3 minutes until the tomatoes start to soften.

6. Season the vegetables with salt and pepper to taste.

7. Add the cooked pasta to the skillet, tossing it with the vegetables to combine.

8. If the pasta seems dry, you can add a splash of the reserved pasta cooking water to moisten it.

9. Sprinkle grated Parmesan cheese over the pasta primavera and stir well to combine.

10. Cook for another 1-2 minutes, or until the cheese is melted and the pasta is heated through.

11. Garnish with thinly sliced fresh basil leaves before serving. Serve the Pasta Primavera hot, optionally with additional grated Parmesan cheese on top.

15. Thai Basil Beef Stir-Fry

Ingredients:
- 1 pound flank steak, thinly sliced against the grain
- 2 tablespoons soy sauce
- 1 tablespoon oyster sauce
- 1 tablespoon fish sauce
- 1 tablespoon brown sugar
- 2 tablespoons vegetable oil
- 4 cloves garlic, minced
- 1 red chili, thinly sliced (adjust to taste)
- 1 bell pepper, thinly sliced
- 1 onion, thinly sliced
- 1 cup fresh basil leaves
- Cooked rice, for serving

Instructions:
1. In a bowl, combine the thinly sliced flank steak with soy sauce, oyster sauce, fish sauce, and brown sugar. Let it marinate for at least 15-20 minutes.

2. Heat vegetable oil in a large skillet over medium-high heat.

3. Add minced garlic and sliced red chili to the skillet. Stir-fry for about 1 minute until fragrant.

4. Add the marinated flank steak to the skillet. Stir-fry for 2-3 minutes until the beef is browned on all sides.

5. Add thinly sliced bell pepper and onion to the skillet. Continue to stir-fry for another 2-3 minutes until the vegetables are tender-crisp.

6. Stir in fresh basil leaves and cook for an additional minute until the basil is wilted.

7. Taste and adjust the seasoning if needed.

8. Remove the skillet from the heat.

9. Serve the Thai Basil Beef Stir-Fry hot, with cooked rice on the side.

Enjoy your delicious and easy single-skillet Thai Basil Beef Stir-Fry!

16. Sausage and Pepper Skillet

Ingredients:
- 1 tablespoon olive oil
- 1 pound Italian sausage, sliced (you can use sweet or spicy, depending on your preference)
- 1 onion, thinly sliced
- 2 bell peppers (any color), thinly sliced
- 2 cloves garlic, minced
- 1 teaspoon Italian seasoning
- Salt and pepper to taste
- Optional: crushed red pepper flakes for added heat
- Chopped fresh parsley for garnish (optional)

Instructions:
1. Heat olive oil in a large skillet over medium-high heat.

2. Add the sliced Italian sausage to the skillet. Cook for about 5-7 minutes, stirring occasionally, until the sausage is browned and cooked through.

3. Add the thinly sliced onion and bell peppers to the skillet. Cook for another 5-7 minutes, or until the vegetables are tender and slightly caramelized.

4. Stir in the minced garlic, Italian seasoning, salt, pepper, and optional crushed red pepper flakes. Cook for an additional 1-2 minutes until the garlic is fragrant.

5. Taste and adjust seasoning if needed.

6. Garnish with chopped fresh parsley, if desired, before serving.

7. Serve the Sausage and Pepper Skillet hot, either on its own or with crusty bread or rolls for sandwiches.

17. Vegetarian Paella

Ingredients:

- 2 tablespoons olive oil
- 1 onion, diced
- 2 cloves garlic, minced
- 1 bell pepper, diced
- 1 zucchini, diced
- 1 cup cherry tomatoes, halved
- 1 cup frozen peas
- 1 1/2 cups Arborio rice
- 3 1/2 cups vegetable broth
- 1 teaspoon smoked paprika
- 1/2 teaspoon saffron threads (optional, for traditional flavor)
- Salt and pepper to taste
- Lemon wedges, for serving
- Chopped fresh parsley for garnish

Instructions:

1. Heat olive oil in a large skillet or paella pan over medium heat.

2. Add diced onion and minced garlic to the skillet. Cook for about 2-3 minutes until softened and fragrant.

3. Stir in diced bell pepper and zucchini. Cook for another 5 minutes until the vegetables are slightly tender.

4. Add Arborio rice to the skillet and stir to coat with the vegetables and oil.

5. Pour vegetable broth into the skillet, then add smoked paprika and saffron threads (if using). Season with salt and pepper to taste. Stir to combine.

6. Bring the mixture to a simmer, then reduce the heat to low. Cover and cook for about 15-20 minutes, stirring occasionally, until the rice is almost tender and most of the liquid is absorbed.

7. Add cherry tomatoes and frozen peas to the skillet, gently stirring them into the rice mixture. Cover and continue to cook for another 5-10 minutes, or until the vegetables are heated through and the rice is fully cooked.

8. Taste and adjust seasoning if needed. Remove the skillet from the heat. Garnish with chopped fresh parsley.

9. Serve the Vegetarian Paella hot, with lemon wedges on the side for squeezing over the paella.

18. Honey Garlic Salmon

Ingredients:
- 4 salmon fillets (about 6 ounces each), skin-on or skinless
- Salt and pepper to taste
- 2 tablespoons olive oil
- 4 cloves garlic, minced
- 1/4 cup soy sauce
- 1/4 cup honey
- 2 tablespoons water
- 1 tablespoon rice vinegar (or white vinegar)
- Optional garnish: sesame seeds, chopped green onions, sliced lemon

Instructions:

1. Season both sides of the salmon fillets with salt and pepper to taste.

2. Heat olive oil in a large skillet over medium-high heat.

3. Place the salmon fillets in the skillet, skin side down if using skin-on fillets. Cook for about 3-4 minutes, or until the salmon easily releases from the skillet and is golden brown on the bottom.

4. Flip the salmon fillets and cook for another 3-4 minutes on the other side, or until they are cooked to your desired level of doneness. Remove the salmon from the skillet and set aside.

5. In the same skillet, add minced garlic and cook for about 1 minute until fragrant.

6. Stir in soy sauce, honey, water, and rice vinegar. Bring the mixture to a simmer, then reduce the heat to low.

7. Return the cooked salmon fillets to the skillet, spooning some of the honey garlic sauce over the top.

8. Cook for another 2-3 minutes, allowing the salmon to absorb some of the sauce and become glazed.

9. Optional: Sprinkle sesame seeds and chopped green onions over the salmon for garnish.

10. Serve the Honey Garlic Salmon hot, optionally with sliced lemon on the side.

Enjoy your delicious and easy single-skillet Honey Garlic Salmon!

19. Cheesy Chicken Enchilada Skillet

Ingredients:
- 1 tablespoon olive oil
- 1 pound boneless, skinless chicken breasts, diced
- Salt and pepper to taste
- 1 small onion, diced
- 1 red bell pepper, diced
- 1 can (10 ounces) red enchilada sauce
- 1 can (4 ounces) diced green chilies
- 1 cup corn kernels (fresh, canned, or frozen)
- 1 cup black beans, drained and rinsed
- 1 cup shredded Mexican blend cheese
- 2 green onions, thinly sliced
- Chopped fresh cilantro, for garnish (optional)
- Tortilla chips or warm tortillas, for serving

Instructions:

1. Heat olive oil in a large skillet over medium heat.

2. Season diced chicken breasts with salt and pepper. Add the seasoned chicken to the skillet and cook for about 5-7 minutes, or until browned and cooked through. Remove chicken from skillet and set aside.

3. In the same skillet, add diced onion and red bell pepper. Cook for 3-4 minutes, until softened.

4. Return cooked chicken to the skillet. Add red enchilada sauce, diced green chilies, corn kernels, and black beans. Stir to combine all ingredients.

5. Allow the mixture to simmer for 2-3 minutes, until heated through.

6. Sprinkle shredded cheese evenly over the top of the skillet.

7. Cover the skillet and cook for another 2-3 minutes, or until the cheese is melted and bubbly.

8. Remove the skillet from heat. Garnish with sliced green onions and chopped fresh cilantro, if desired.

9. Serve the Cheesy Chicken Enchilada Skillet hot, with tortilla chips or warm tortillas on the side.

20. Lemon Garlic Butter Shrimp and Broccoli

Ingredients:
- 1 pound large shrimp, peeled and deveined
- Salt and pepper to taste
- 2 tablespoons olive oil
- 4 cloves garlic, minced
- 1 head broccoli, cut into florets
- Zest and juice of 1 lemon
- 4 tablespoons unsalted butter
- Optional: Crushed red pepper flakes for heat
- Fresh chopped parsley for garnish

Instructions:

1. Season the shrimp with salt and pepper to taste.

2. Heat olive oil in a large skillet over medium-high heat.

3. Add minced garlic to the skillet and sauté for about 1 minute until fragrant.

4. Add the seasoned shrimp to the skillet and cook for 2-3 minutes on each side until pink and cooked through. Remove the shrimp from the skillet and set aside.

5. In the same skillet, add broccoli florets. Cook for about 4-5 minutes, stirring occasionally, until they are bright green and slightly tender.

6. Add lemon zest and juice to the skillet, along with unsalted butter. Stir until the butter is melted and coats the broccoli.

7. Return the cooked shrimp to the skillet and toss to coat with the lemon garlic butter sauce.

8. If desired, add crushed red pepper flakes for heat and extra flavor.

9. Cook for another 1-2 minutes until everything is heated through.

10. Garnish with fresh chopped parsley before serving.

11. Serve the Lemon Garlic Butter Shrimp and Broccoli hot, optionally with cooked rice or pasta on the side.

Enjoy your delicious and easy single-skillet Lemon Garlic Butter Shrimp and Broccoli!

21. Mexican Quinoa

Ingredients:
- 1 tablespoon olive oil
- 1 small onion, diced
- 2 cloves garlic, minced
- 1 bell pepper, diced
- 1 cup quinoa, rinsed and drained
- 1 can (15 ounces) black beans, drained and rinsed
- 1 can (15 ounces) diced tomatoes
- 1 cup vegetable broth or water
- 1 teaspoon chili powder
- 1 teaspoon ground cumin
- 1/2 teaspoon paprika
- Salt and pepper to taste
- Optional toppings: chopped fresh cilantro, sliced avocado, diced tomatoes, shredded cheese, sour cream, lime wedges

Instructions:
1. Heat olive oil in a large skillet over medium heat.

2. Add diced onion and minced garlic to the skillet. Cook for 2-3 minutes until softened and fragrant.

3. Stir in diced bell pepper and cook for another 2-3 minutes until slightly softened.

4. Add rinsed quinoa to the skillet. Cook for 1-2 minutes, stirring frequently, until the quinoa is lightly toasted.

5. Stir in drained and rinsed black beans, diced tomatoes, vegetable broth (or water), chili powder, ground cumin, paprika, salt, and pepper.

6. Bring the mixture to a simmer, then reduce the heat to low.

7. Cover the skillet and let it simmer for about 15-20 minutes, or until the quinoa is cooked and the liquid is absorbed. Stir occasionally to prevent sticking.

8. Once the quinoa is cooked, taste and adjust seasoning if needed.

9. Remove the skillet from the heat and fluff the quinoa with a fork.

10. Serve the Mexican Quinoa hot, optionally topped with chopped fresh cilantro, sliced avocado, diced tomatoes, shredded cheese, sour cream, and lime wedges

22. Skillet Lasagna

Ingredients:
- 1 tablespoon olive oil
- 1 onion, diced
- 2 cloves garlic, minced
- 1 pound ground beef or Italian sausage
- 1 can (14.5 ounces) diced tomatoes
- 1 can (8 ounces) tomato sauce
- 1 teaspoon dried basil
- 1 teaspoon dried oregano
- Salt and pepper to taste
- 2 cups uncooked bowtie pasta (farfalle) or any other short pasta
- 2 cups water or beef broth
- 1 cup shredded mozzarella cheese
- 1/2 cup ricotta cheese
- Chopped fresh parsley, for garnish (optional)

Instructions:

1. Heat olive oil in a large skillet over medium heat.

2. Add diced onion and minced garlic to the skillet. Cook for 2-3 minutes until softened and fragrant.

3. Add ground beef or Italian sausage to the skillet. Cook, breaking up the meat with a spoon, until browned and cooked through.

4. Stir in diced tomatoes, tomato sauce, dried basil, dried oregano, salt, and pepper. Mix well to combine.

5. Add uncooked pasta to the skillet, spreading it out in an even layer.

6. Pour water or beef broth over the pasta, making sure it's completely covered.

7. Bring the mixture to a simmer, then reduce the heat to low.

8. Cover the skillet and let it simmer for about 12-15 minutes, or until the pasta is cooked and most of the liquid is absorbed, stirring occasionally.

9. Once the pasta is cooked, dollop ricotta cheese over the top of the skillet lasagna.

10. Sprinkle shredded mozzarella cheese over the skillet lasagna.

11. Cover the skillet and let it sit for a few minutes until the cheese is melted and bubbly.

12. Garnish with chopped fresh parsley, if desired, before serving.

13. Serve the Skillet Lasagna hot, straight from the skillet.

23. Tofu and Vegetable Stir-Fry

Ingredients:

- 14 ounces firm tofu, drained and pressed
- 2 tablespoons soy sauce
- 1 tablespoon sesame oil
- 2 tablespoons olive oil or vegetable oil, divided
- 2 cloves garlic, minced
- 1 tablespoon grated ginger
- 1 bell pepper, thinly sliced
- 1 carrot, julienned or thinly sliced
- 1 cup broccoli florets
- 1 cup snap peas, trimmed
- 1 cup sliced mushrooms
- Salt and pepper to taste
- Cooked rice or noodles, for serving
- Optional garnishes: sliced green onions, sesame seeds, chopped cilantro

Instructions:

1. Cut the pressed tofu into cubes.

2. In a small bowl, mix together soy sauce and sesame oil. Add tofu cubes to the bowl and gently toss to coat. Let it marinate for about 10-15 minutes.

3. Heat 1 tablespoon of olive oil in a large skillet over medium-high heat.

4. Add marinated tofu cubes to the skillet in a single layer. Cook for about 3-4 minutes on each side until golden brown and crispy. Remove tofu from the skillet and set aside.

5. In the same skillet, add the remaining tablespoon of olive oil.

6. Add minced garlic and grated ginger to the skillet. Cook for about 1 minute until fragrant.

7. Add thinly sliced bell pepper, julienned carrot, broccoli florets, snap peas, and sliced mushrooms to the skillet. Stir-fry for about 5-6 minutes until the vegetables are tender-crisp.

8. Season the vegetables with salt and pepper to taste.

9. Return the cooked tofu to the skillet and gently toss everything together to combine.

10. Cook for another 1-2 minutes until everything is heated through.

11. Serve the Tofu and Vegetable Stir-Fry hot, over cooked rice or noodles.

12. Garnish with sliced green onions, sesame seeds, and chopped cilantro if desired.

Enjoy your delicious and easy single-skillet Tofu and Vegetable Stir-Fry!

24. One-Pot Lemon Herb Chicken and Rice

Ingredients:

- 4 bone-in, skin-on chicken thighs
- Salt and pepper to taste
- 2 tablespoons olive oil
- 1 onion, diced
- 2 cloves garlic, minced
- 1 cup long-grain white rice
- 2 cups chicken broth
- Zest and juice of 1 lemon
- 1 teaspoon dried thyme
- 1 teaspoon dried rosemary
- 1/2 teaspoon dried oregano
- 1 cup frozen peas
- Fresh parsley, chopped, for garnish (optional)

Instructions:

1. Season the chicken thighs with salt and pepper to taste.

2. Heat olive oil in a large skillet over medium-high heat.

3. Add the chicken thighs to the skillet, skin side down. Cook for about 5-6 minutes on each side until golden brown. Remove the chicken from the skillet and set aside.

4. In the same skillet, add diced onion and minced garlic. Cook for 2-3 minutes until softened and fragrant.

5. Stir in the rice and cook for another 1-2 minutes, stirring occasionally, until the rice is lightly toasted.

6. Pour in the chicken broth, lemon zest, lemon juice, dried thyme, dried rosemary, and dried oregano. Stir to combine.

7. Return the cooked chicken thighs to the skillet, nestling them into the rice mixture.

8. Bring the mixture to a simmer, then reduce the heat to low. Cover the skillet and let it simmer for about 20-25 minutes, or until the rice is cooked and the chicken is cooked through.

9. Add frozen peas to the skillet during the last 5 minutes of cooking, stirring them into the rice mixture.

10. Taste and adjust seasoning if needed.

11. Garnish with chopped fresh parsley, if desired, before serving.

12. Serve the One-Pot Lemon Herb Chicken and Rice hot, straight from the skillet.

25. Zucchini Noodles with Pesto and Cherry Tomatoes

Ingredients:

- 4 medium zucchini
- 1 tablespoon olive oil
- 1 cup cherry tomatoes, halved
- Salt and pepper to taste
- 1/4 cup pesto sauce (store-bought or homemade)
- Grated Parmesan cheese, for garnish (optional)
- Fresh basil leaves, torn, for garnish (optional)

Instructions:

1. Using a spiralizer or vegetable peeler, create zucchini noodles (also known as zoodles) from the zucchini. Set aside.

2. Heat olive oil in a large skillet over medium heat.

3. Add the halved cherry tomatoes to the skillet. Cook for about 2-3 minutes until they start to soften.

4. Add the zucchini noodles to the skillet. Toss with the cherry tomatoes and cook for another 2-3 minutes until the zucchini noodles are just tender but still slightly crisp.

5. Season the zucchini noodles and cherry tomatoes with salt and pepper to taste.

6. Stir in the pesto sauce, making sure to coat the zucchini noodles and cherry tomatoes evenly.

7. Cook for another 1-2 minutes until everything is heated through.

8. Remove the skillet from the heat.

9. Serve the Zucchini Noodles with Pesto and Cherry Tomatoes hot, optionally garnished with grated Parmesan cheese and torn fresh basil leaves.

Enjoy your delicious and easy single-skillet Zucchini Noodles with Pesto and Cherry Tomatoes!

26. Creamy Mushroom Risotto

Ingredients:

- 1 tablespoon olive oil
- 2 tablespoons butter, divided
- 1 small onion, finely chopped
- 2 cloves garlic, minced
- 8 ounces mushrooms (such as cremini or button), sliced
- 1 cup Arborio rice
- 1/2 cup dry white wine (optional)
- 4 cups vegetable or chicken broth, warmed
- 1/2 cup grated Parmesan cheese
- Salt and pepper to taste
- Chopped fresh parsley, for garnish (optional)

Instructions:

1. In a large skillet, heat the olive oil and 1 tablespoon of butter over medium heat.

2. Add the chopped onion and cook for 2-3 minutes until softened.

3. Stir in the minced garlic and cook for an additional minute until fragrant.

4. Add the sliced mushrooms to the skillet and cook for 5-7 minutes until they release their moisture and start to brown. Remove some of the mushrooms and set them aside for garnish if desired.

5. Stir in the Arborio rice and cook for 1-2 minutes, stirring constantly, until the rice is lightly toasted.

6. If using, pour in the white wine and cook until it is mostly absorbed by the rice, stirring frequently.

7. Begin adding the warmed broth to the skillet, about 1/2 cup at a time, stirring frequently and allowing the liquid to be absorbed before adding more. Continue this process until the rice is creamy and cooked through, which should take about 20-25 minutes. You may not need to use all of the broth.

8. Once the rice is cooked to your desired consistency, stir in the remaining tablespoon of butter and grated Parmesan cheese. Season with salt and pepper to taste.

9. If desired, garnish the creamy mushroom risotto with the reserved cooked mushrooms and chopped fresh parsley.

10. Serve the risotto hot, optionally with additional grated Parmesan cheese on top.

27. Blackened Tilapia

Ingredients:
- 4 tilapia fillets
- 2 tablespoons olive oil
- 1 tablespoon paprika
- 1 teaspoon garlic powder
- 1 teaspoon onion powder
- 1 teaspoon dried thyme
- 1 teaspoon dried oregano
- 1/2 teaspoon cayenne pepper (adjust to taste)
- 1/2 teaspoon salt
- 1/4 teaspoon black pepper
- 1 lemon, cut into wedges for serving
- Chopped fresh parsley or cilantro for garnish (optional)

Instructions:
1. In a small bowl, mix together paprika, garlic powder, onion powder, dried thyme, dried oregano, cayenne pepper, salt, and black pepper to make the blackening seasoning.

2. Pat the tilapia fillets dry with paper towels.

3. Rub both sides of each tilapia fillet with the blackening seasoning mixture, ensuring they are evenly coated.

4. Heat olive oil in a large skillet over medium-high heat.

5. Once the skillet is hot, carefully add the seasoned tilapia fillets to the skillet.

6. Cook the tilapia for about 3-4 minutes on each side, or until they are cooked through and blackened on the outside.

7. Remove the skillet from the heat.

8. Squeeze fresh lemon juice over the blackened tilapia fillets.

9. Garnish with chopped fresh parsley or cilantro, if desired.

10. Serve the Blackened Tilapia hot, with lemon wedges on the side for additional flavor.

28. Pineapple Chicken Stir-Fry

Ingredients:
- 1 pound boneless, skinless chicken breasts, cut into bite-sized pieces
- Salt and pepper to taste
- 2 tablespoons vegetable oil, divided
- 1 red bell pepper, sliced
- 1 green bell pepper, sliced
- 1 small onion, sliced
- 1 cup pineapple chunks (fresh or canned)
- 3 cloves garlic, minced
- 1/4 cup soy sauce
- 2 tablespoons honey
- 1 tablespoon rice vinegar
- 1 tablespoon cornstarch
- Cooked rice, for serving
- Optional garnish: chopped green onions, sesame seeds

Instructions:

1. Season the chicken pieces with salt and pepper to taste.

2. Heat 1 tablespoon of vegetable oil in a large skillet over medium-high heat.

3. Add the seasoned chicken pieces to the skillet and cook for 5-6 minutes, stirring occasionally, until browned and cooked through. Remove the chicken from the skillet and set aside.

4. In the same skillet, add the remaining tablespoon of vegetable oil.

5. Add the sliced red and green bell peppers, along with the sliced onion, to the skillet. Cook for 3-4 minutes until the vegetables are tender-crisp.

6. Stir in the pineapple chunks and minced garlic. Cook for an additional 1-2 minutes until the garlic is fragrant.

7. In a small bowl, whisk together soy sauce, honey, rice vinegar, and cornstarch until smooth.

8. Pour the sauce mixture into the skillet with the vegetables and pineapple. Stir well to combine.

9. Return the cooked chicken to the skillet and toss everything together until the chicken is coated with the sauce.

10. Cook for another 2-3 minutes, stirring occasionally, until the sauce has thickened and everything is heated through.

11. Serve the Pineapple Chicken Stir-Fry hot, over cooked rice. Garnish with chopped green onions and sesame seeds if desired.

29. Teriyaki Tofu and Vegetable Stir-Fry

Ingredients:
- 1 block (14-16 ounces) firm tofu, pressed and cubed
  - 1/4 cup soy sauce
  - 2 tablespoons honey or maple syrup
  - 2 tablespoons rice vinegar
  - 1 tablespoon sesame oil
  - 2 cloves garlic, minced
  - 1 teaspoon grated ginger
  - 1 tablespoon cornstarch
  - 2 tablespoons water
- 2 tablespoons vegetable oil, divided
- 1 bell pepper, thinly sliced
- 1 carrot, julienned or thinly sliced
- 1 cup broccoli florets
- 1 cup snap peas or snow peas, trimmed
- Cooked rice or noodles, for serving
- Optional garnish: sesame seeds, sliced green onions

Instructions:

1. In a small bowl, whisk together soy sauce, honey (or maple syrup), rice vinegar, sesame oil, minced garlic, and grated ginger to make the teriyaki sauce. Set aside.

2. In another small bowl, mix together cornstarch and water to make a slurry. Set aside.

3. Heat 1 tablespoon of vegetable oil in a large skillet over medium-high heat.

4. Add the cubed tofu to the skillet in a single layer. Cook for about 5-6 minutes, stirring occasionally, until the tofu is golden brown and crispy on all sides. Remove the tofu from the skillet and set aside.

5. In the same skillet, add the remaining tablespoon of vegetable oil.

6. Add sliced bell pepper, julienned carrot, broccoli florets, and snap peas to the skillet. Stir-fry for about 4-5 minutes until the vegetables are tender-crisp.

7. Return the cooked tofu to the skillet.

8. Give the teriyaki sauce a quick stir to recombine, then pour it over the tofu and vegetables in the skillet.

9. Pour the cornstarch slurry over the tofu and vegetables. Stir well to combine, allowing the sauce to thicken.

10. Cook for another 1-2 minutes until the sauce coats everything evenly.

11. Serve the Teriyaki Tofu and Vegetable Stir-Fry hot, over cooked rice or noodles. Garnish with sesame seeds and sliced green onions if desired.

30. Italian Sausage and Peppers Pasta

Ingredients:
- 8 ounces pasta (such as penne or rigatoni)
- 1 tablespoon olive oil
- 1 pound Italian sausage (sweet or spicy), casings removed
- 1 onion, thinly sliced
- 1 red bell pepper, thinly sliced
- 1 green bell pepper, thinly sliced
- 3 cloves garlic, minced
- 1 can (14.5 ounces) diced tomatoes
- 1 teaspoon dried oregano
- 1/2 teaspoon dried basil
- Salt and pepper to taste
- Grated Parmesan cheese, for serving
- Chopped fresh parsley, for garnish (optional)

Instructions:
1. Cook the pasta according to package instructions until al dente. Drain and set aside.

2. In a large skillet, heat the olive oil over medium-high heat.

3. Add the Italian sausage to the skillet, breaking it up with a spoon. Cook for 5-6 minutes until browned and cooked through.

4. Add the thinly sliced onion and bell peppers to the skillet. Cook for another 4-5 minutes until the vegetables are softened.

5. Stir in the minced garlic and cook for an additional minute until fragrant.

6. Add the diced tomatoes (with their juices) to the skillet. Stir in the dried oregano and dried basil. Season with salt and pepper to taste.

7. Bring the mixture to a simmer and let it cook for 5-7 minutes until slightly thickened, stirring occasionally.

8. Add the cooked pasta to the skillet. Toss everything together until the pasta is coated with the sauce.

9. Cook for another 1-2 minutes until everything is heated through.

10. Serve the Italian Sausage and Peppers Pasta hot, topped with grated Parmesan cheese and chopped fresh parsley if desired.

31. One-Pan Garlic Butter Salmon with Asparagus

Ingredients:

- 4 salmon fillets
- Salt and pepper to taste
- 2 tablespoons olive oil
- 2 tablespoons butter
- 4 cloves garlic, minced
- 1 pound asparagus, trimmed
- Juice of 1/2 lemon
- Lemon slices for garnish (optional)
- Chopped fresh parsley for garnish (optional)

Instructions:

1. Season both sides of the salmon fillets with salt and pepper to taste.

2. Heat olive oil in a large skillet over medium-high heat.

3. Place the salmon fillets in the skillet, skin side down if they have skin. Cook for about 4-5 minutes until nicely browned on the bottom.

4. Flip the salmon fillets and add butter and minced garlic to the skillet. Cook for another 3-4 minutes, spooning the garlic butter sauce over the salmon, until the salmon is cooked to your desired level of doneness.

5. Remove the salmon from the skillet and set aside.

6. In the same skillet, add the trimmed asparagus. Cook for about 4-5 minutes, stirring occasionally, until the asparagus is tender-crisp.

7. Squeeze lemon juice over the asparagus and toss to coat.

8. Return the cooked salmon to the skillet, arranging it among the asparagus.

9. Garnish with lemon slices and chopped fresh parsley, if desired.

10. Serve the One-Pan Garlic Butter Salmon with Asparagus hot, optionally with cooked rice or quinoa on the side.

32. Tex-Mex Beef and Rice Skillet

Ingredients:
- 1 tablespoon olive oil
- 1 pound ground beef
- 1 onion, diced
- 1 bell pepper, diced
- 2 cloves garlic, minced
- 1 cup long-grain white rice
- 1 can (15 ounces) black beans, drained and rinsed
- 1 can (14.5 ounces) diced tomatoes
- 1 cup corn kernels (fresh, canned, or frozen)
- 1 cup beef broth
- 1 tablespoon chili powder
- 1 teaspoon ground cumin
- Salt and pepper to taste
- Optional toppings: shredded cheese, diced avocado, sour cream, chopped cilantro, sliced jalapeños

Instructions:

1. Heat olive oil in a large skillet over medium-high heat.

2. Add ground beef to the skillet and cook, breaking it up with a spoon, until browned and cooked through.

3. Add diced onion, diced bell pepper, and minced garlic to the skillet. Cook for 2-3 minutes until the vegetables are softened.

4. Stir in long-grain white rice and cook for another 1-2 minutes, stirring occasionally, until the rice is lightly toasted.

5. Add drained and rinsed black beans, diced tomatoes, corn kernels, beef broth, chili powder, and ground cumin to the skillet. Stir well to combine.

6. Season with salt and pepper to taste.

7. Bring the mixture to a simmer, then reduce the heat to low.

8. Cover the skillet and let it simmer for about 15-20 minutes, or until the rice is cooked and most of the liquid is absorbed, stirring occasionally.

9. Once the rice is cooked, taste and adjust seasoning if needed.

10. Serve the Tex-Mex Beef and Rice Skillet hot, topped with shredded cheese, diced avocado, sour cream, chopped cilantro, and sliced jalapeños if desired.

Enjoy your delicious and easy single-skillet Tex-Mex Beef and Rice Skillet!

33. Coconut Curry Shrimp

Ingredients:

- 1 tablespoon vegetable oil
- 1 onion, diced
- 2 cloves garlic, minced
- 1 tablespoon grated ginger
- 1 red bell pepper, sliced
- 1 yellow bell pepper, sliced
- 1 can (14 ounces) coconut milk
- 2 tablespoons red curry paste
- 1 tablespoon fish sauce
- 1 tablespoon brown sugar
- 1 pound large shrimp, peeled and deveined
- Salt and pepper to taste
- Juice of 1 lime
- Cooked rice, for serving
- Chopped fresh cilantro, for garnish

Instructions:

1. Heat vegetable oil in a large skillet over medium heat.

2. Add diced onion, minced garlic, and grated ginger to the skillet. Cook for 2-3 minutes until fragrant.

3. Add sliced red bell pepper and yellow bell pepper to the skillet. Cook for another 3-4 minutes until the peppers are slightly softened.

4. Pour in coconut milk, red curry paste, fish sauce, and brown sugar. Stir well to combine.

5. Bring the mixture to a simmer and let it cook for 5 minutes, stirring occasionally.

6. Season the shrimp with salt and pepper to taste.

7. Add the seasoned shrimp to the skillet. Cook for 3-4 minutes until the shrimp are pink and cooked through.

8. Squeeze the juice of 1 lime over the shrimp curry.

9. Taste and adjust seasoning if needed.

10. Serve the Coconut Curry Shrimp hot, over cooked rice. Garnish with chopped fresh cilantro before serving.

34. Skillet BBQ Chicken and Potatoes

Ingredients:
- 4 boneless, skinless chicken breasts
- Salt and pepper to taste
- 2 tablespoons olive oil
- 4 medium potatoes, diced into cubes
- 1 onion, diced
- 1 bell pepper, diced
- 1 cup barbecue sauce
- 1/2 cup chicken broth or water
- Optional: chopped fresh parsley or green onions for garnish

Instructions:

1. Season both sides of the chicken breasts with salt and pepper to taste.

2. Heat olive oil in a large skillet over medium-high heat.

3. Add the seasoned chicken breasts to the skillet. Cook for about 5-6 minutes on each side until golden brown and cooked through. Remove the chicken from the skillet and set aside.

4. In the same skillet, add diced potatoes. Cook for about 5-7 minutes, stirring occasionally, until they start to brown and become tender.

5. Add diced onion and bell pepper to the skillet with the potatoes. Cook for another 3-4 minutes until the vegetables are softened.

6. Return the cooked chicken breasts to the skillet, nestling them among the potatoes and vegetables.

7. In a small bowl, mix together barbecue sauce and chicken broth (or water). Pour the sauce mixture over the chicken, potatoes, and vegetables in the skillet.

8. Reduce the heat to medium-low. Cover the skillet and let it simmer for about 8-10 minutes, stirring occasionally, until everything is heated through and the flavors are melded together.

9. Taste and adjust seasoning if needed.

10. Serve the Skillet BBQ Chicken and Potatoes hot, optionally garnished with chopped fresh parsley or green onions.

Enjoy your delicious and easy single-skillet Skillet BBQ Chicken and Potatoes!

35. Ratatouille

Ingredients:
- 2 tablespoons olive oil
- 1 onion, diced
- 3 cloves garlic, minced
- 1 eggplant, diced
- 2 zucchini, diced
- 1 bell pepper, diced
- 2 tomatoes, diced
- 1 teaspoon dried thyme
- 1 teaspoon dried oregano
- Salt and pepper to taste
- Fresh basil leaves, chopped, for garnish

Instructions:
1. Heat olive oil in a large skillet over medium heat.

2. Add diced onion and minced garlic to the skillet. Cook for 2-3 minutes until softened and fragrant.

3. Add diced eggplant to the skillet. Cook for about 5 minutes, stirring occasionally, until the eggplant starts to soften.

4. Stir in diced zucchini and diced bell pepper. Cook for another 5 minutes until the vegetables are tender-crisp.

5. Add diced tomatoes to the skillet, along with dried thyme and dried oregano. Season with salt and pepper to taste.

6. Stir well to combine all the ingredients.

7. Reduce the heat to low, cover the skillet, and let the ratatouille simmer for about 15-20 minutes, stirring occasionally, until all the vegetables are cooked through and flavors are melded together.

8. Taste and adjust seasoning if needed.

9. Serve the Ratatouille hot, garnished with chopped fresh basil leaves.

Enjoy your delicious and easy single-skillet Ratatouille!

36. Crispy Tofu Stir-Fry

Ingredients:

- 1 block (14-16 ounces) firm tofu
- 2 tablespoons cornstarch
- Salt and pepper to taste
- 2 tablespoons vegetable oil, divided
- 2 cloves garlic, minced
- 1 tablespoon grated ginger
- 1 bell pepper, sliced
- 1 carrot, julienned or thinly sliced
- 1 cup broccoli florets
- 1 cup snap peas or snow peas, trimmed
- 1/4 cup soy sauce
- 2 tablespoons rice vinegar
- 1 tablespoon honey or maple syrup
- Cooked rice or noodles, for serving
- Optional garnish: sliced green onions, sesame seeds

Instructions:

1. Press the tofu to remove excess moisture: Wrap the tofu block in a clean kitchen towel or paper towels and place something heavy on top (like a cast iron skillet or a few heavy books). Let it press for about 15-20 minutes.

2. Once pressed, cut the tofu into bite-sized cubes.

3. Place the tofu cubes in a bowl and toss with cornstarch, salt, and pepper until evenly coated.

4. Heat 1 tablespoon of vegetable oil in a large skillet over medium-high heat.

5. Add the coated tofu cubes to the skillet in a single layer. Cook for about 3-4 minutes on each side until golden brown and crispy. Remove the tofu from the skillet and set aside.

6. In the same skillet, add the remaining tablespoon of vegetable oil.

7. Add minced garlic and grated ginger to the skillet. Cook for about 1 minute until fragrant.

8. Add sliced bell pepper, julienned carrot, broccoli florets, and snap peas to the skillet. Stir-fry for about 4-5 minutes until the vegetables are tender-crisp.

9. In a small bowl, whisk together soy sauce, rice vinegar, and honey (or maple syrup). Return the cooked tofu to the skillet.

11. Pour the sauce mixture over the tofu and vegetables in the skillet. Stir well to combine.

12. Cook for another 1-2 minutes until everything is heated through and the sauce coats everything evenly.

13. Serve the Crispy Tofu Stir-Fry hot, over cooked rice or noodles. Garnish with sliced green onions and sesame seeds if desired. Enjoy your delicious and easy single-skillet Crispy Tofu Stir-Fry!

37. Mediterranean Chickpea Skillet

Ingredients:

- 2 tablespoons olive oil
- 1 onion, diced
- 3 cloves garlic, minced
- 1 red bell pepper, diced
- 1 yellow bell pepper, diced
- 1 zucchini, diced
- 1 teaspoon dried oregano
- 1 teaspoon dried basil
- 1/2 teaspoon smoked paprika
- Salt and pepper to taste
- 1 can (15 ounces) chickpeas, drained and rinsed
- 1 can (14.5 ounces) diced tomatoes
- 1/2 cup pitted Kalamata olives, halved
- 2 tablespoons capers, drained
- Juice of 1 lemon
- Crumbled feta cheese, for serving (optional)
- Chopped fresh parsley or basil, for garnish

Instructions:

1. Heat olive oil in a large skillet over medium heat.

2. Add diced onion and minced garlic to the skillet. Cook for 2-3 minutes until softened and fragrant.

3. Add diced red bell pepper, yellow bell pepper, and diced zucchini to the skillet. Cook for about 5 minutes until the vegetables start to soften.

4. Stir in dried oregano, dried basil, smoked paprika, salt, and pepper. Cook for another minute until fragrant.

5. Add drained and rinsed chickpeas, diced tomatoes (with their juices), halved Kalamata olives, and drained capers to the skillet. Stir well to combine.

6. Reduce the heat to low, cover the skillet, and let it simmer for about 10-15 minutes, stirring occasionally, until the flavors are melded together and the vegetables are cooked through.

7. Squeeze the juice of 1 lemon over the chickpea skillet and stir to combine. Taste and adjust seasoning if needed.

9. Serve the Mediterranean Chickpea Skillet hot, optionally topped with crumbled feta cheese and chopped fresh parsley or basil. Enjoy your delicious and easy single-skillet Mediterranean Chickpea Skillet!

38. Creamy Lemon Chicken Piccata

Ingredients:
- 4 boneless, skinless chicken breasts
- Salt and pepper to taste
- 2 tablespoons all-purpose flour
- 2 tablespoons olive oil
- 3 cloves garlic, minced
- 1/2 cup chicken broth
- 1/4 cup fresh lemon juice
- Zest of 1 lemon
- 1/4 cup heavy cream
- 2 tablespoons capers, drained
- 2 tablespoons unsalted butter
- Chopped fresh parsley, for garnish
- Lemon slices, for garnish

Instructions:
1. Season both sides of the chicken breasts with salt and pepper. Dredge each chicken breast in flour, shaking off any excess.

2. Heat olive oil in a large skillet over medium-high heat.

3. Add the chicken breasts to the skillet and cook for about 4-5 minutes on each side, or until golden brown and cooked through. Remove the chicken from the skillet and set aside.

4. In the same skillet, add minced garlic and cook for about 1 minute, until fragrant.

5. Pour chicken broth and lemon juice into the skillet, scraping up any browned bits from the bottom of the pan. Allow the mixture to simmer for about 2-3 minutes.

6. Stir in lemon zest, heavy cream, and capers. Let the sauce simmer for another 2-3 minutes until slightly thickened.

7. Add unsalted butter to the skillet and stir until melted and incorporated into the sauce.

8. Return the cooked chicken breasts to the skillet, spooning the sauce over the top. Let the chicken simmer in the sauce for an additional 2-3 minutes to heat through.

9. Garnish with chopped fresh parsley and lemon slices before serving.

10. Serve the Creamy Lemon Chicken Piccata hot, with your choice of side dishes like pasta, rice, or vegetables.

39. Szechuan Beef and Broccoli

Ingredients:

- 1 pound flank steak, thinly sliced against the grain
- 2 tablespoons soy sauce
- 1 tablespoon cornstarch
- 1 tablespoon vegetable oil
- 3 cloves garlic, minced
- 1 teaspoon grated ginger
- 1/4 cup soy sauce
- 2 tablespoons hoisin sauce
- 1 tablespoon rice vinegar
- 1 tablespoon brown sugar
- 1 teaspoon sesame oil
- 1/2 teaspoon crushed red pepper flakes (adjust to taste)
- 2 cups broccoli florets
- Cooked rice, for serving
- Optional garnish: sliced green onions, sesame seeds

Instructions:

1. In a bowl, combine thinly sliced flank steak with 2 tablespoons of soy sauce and cornstarch. Mix well to coat the beef evenly. Let it marinate for about 15-20 minutes.

2. Heat vegetable oil in a large skillet over medium-high heat.

3. Add minced garlic and grated ginger to the skillet. Cook for about 1 minute until fragrant.

4. Add the marinated beef slices to the skillet in a single layer. Cook for about 2-3 minutes on each side until browned and cooked through. Remove the beef from the skillet and set aside.

5. In the same skillet, add soy sauce, hoisin sauce, rice vinegar, brown sugar, sesame oil, and crushed red pepper flakes. Stir well to combine.

6. Add broccoli florets to the skillet. Cook for about 4-5 minutes, stirring occasionally, until the broccoli is tender-crisp.

7. Return the cooked beef to the skillet. Toss everything together until the beef is coated with the sauce.

8. Cook for another 1-2 minutes until everything is heated through.

9. Serve the Szechuan Beef and Broccoli hot, over cooked rice.

10. Garnish with sliced green onions and sesame seeds if desired.

Enjoy your delicious and easy single-skillet Szechuan Beef and Broccoli!

40. One-Pan Pesto Chicken and Vegetables

Ingredients:
- 4 boneless, skinless chicken breasts
- Salt and pepper to taste
- 2 tablespoons olive oil
- 1 red bell pepper, sliced
- 1 yellow bell pepper, sliced
- 1 zucchini, sliced
- 1 yellow squash, sliced
- 1/2 cup cherry tomatoes, halved
- 1/4 cup basil pesto
- 1/4 cup grated Parmesan cheese
- Fresh basil leaves, for garnish (optional)

Instructions:

1. Season both sides of the chicken breasts with salt and pepper.

2. Heat olive oil in a large skillet over medium-high heat.

3. Add the chicken breasts to the skillet and cook for about 5-6 minutes on each side until golden brown and cooked through. Remove the chicken from the skillet and set aside.

4. In the same skillet, add sliced red bell pepper, yellow bell pepper, zucchini, yellow squash, and cherry tomatoes. Cook for about 5-7 minutes, stirring occasionally, until the vegetables are tender-crisp.

5. Return the cooked chicken breasts to the skillet, placing them on top of the cooked vegetables.

6. Spoon basil pesto over each chicken breast, spreading it evenly.

7. Sprinkle grated Parmesan cheese over the chicken and vegetables.

8. Cover the skillet and let it simmer for another 2-3 minutes, allowing the flavors to meld together.

9. Garnish with fresh basil leaves if desired.

10. Serve the One-Pan Pesto Chicken and Vegetables hot, optionally with cooked pasta or rice on the side.

Enjoy your delicious and easy single-skillet One-Pan Pesto Chicken and Vegetables!

41. Quinoa Stuffed Peppers

Ingredients:

- 4 large bell peppers (any color), halved and seeds removed
- 1 cup quinoa, rinsed
- 2 cups vegetable broth or water
- 1 tablespoon olive oil
- 1 onion, diced
- 2 cloves garlic, minced
- 1 cup diced tomatoes (fresh or canned)
- 1 teaspoon dried oregano
- 1 zucchini, diced
- 1 carrot, diced
- 1 teaspoon dried basil
- Salt and pepper to taste
- 1 cup shredded cheese (such as mozzarella or cheddar)
- Chopped fresh parsley or basil, for garnish

Instructions:

1. Preheat your oven to 375°F (190°C). Place the halved bell peppers in a baking dish, cut side up.

2. In a skillet, combine quinoa and vegetable broth (or water). Bring to a boil, then reduce heat to low, cover, and simmer for about 15 minutes, or until the quinoa is cooked and the liquid is absorbed. Remove from heat and set aside.

3. In the same skillet, heat olive oil over medium heat. Add diced onion and cook for 2-3 minutes until softened.

4. Add minced garlic, diced zucchini, and diced carrot to the skillet. Cook for another 3-4 minutes until the vegetables are tender.

5. Stir in diced tomatoes, dried oregano, dried basil, cooked quinoa, salt, and pepper. Cook for an additional 2-3 minutes to combine all the flavors.

6. Spoon the quinoa and vegetable mixture into the halved bell peppers, pressing down gently to fill each pepper.

7. Sprinkle shredded cheese over the stuffed peppers.

8. Cover the baking dish with aluminum foil and bake in the preheated oven for about 25-30 minutes, or until the peppers are tender and the cheese is melted and bubbly.

9. Remove from the oven and let the stuffed peppers cool for a few minutes.

10. Garnish with chopped fresh parsley or basil before serving. Serve the Quinoa Stuffed Peppers hot, optionally with a side of salad.

Enjoy your delicious and easy single-skillet Quinoa Stuffed Peppers!

42. Skillet Macaroni and Cheese

Ingredients:

- **2** cups elbow macaroni
- 2 tablespoons butter
- 2 tablespoons all-purpose flour
- 2 cups milk
- 2 cups shredded cheddar cheese (or your favorite cheese blend)
- Salt and pepper to taste
- Optional add-ins: cooked bacon bits, diced ham, peas, diced bell peppers, etc.
- Optional toppings: bread crumbs, chopped parsley, grated Parmesan cheese

Instructions:

1. Cook the elbow macaroni according to the package instructions until al dente. Drain and set aside.

2. In the same skillet, melt butter over medium heat.

3. Stir in all-purpose flour and cook for about 1-2 minutes to make a roux, stirring constantly.

4. Gradually pour in milk, whisking constantly to avoid lumps. Cook until the mixture thickens, about 3-4 minutes.

5. Reduce the heat to low. Stir in shredded cheddar cheese until melted and smooth.

6. Season the cheese sauce with salt and pepper to taste.

7. If using any optional add-ins, stir them into the cheese sauce at this point.

8. Add the cooked macaroni to the skillet with the cheese sauce. Stir until the macaroni is evenly coated with the sauce.

9. If desired, sprinkle bread crumbs, chopped parsley, or grated Parmesan cheese over the top.

10. Cover the skillet and let it cook for another 2-3 minutes until heated through.

11. Serve the Skillet Macaroni and Cheese hot, straight from the skillet.

Enjoy your delicious and easy single-skillet Skillet Macaroni and Cheese!

43. Honey Mustard Glazed Salmon

Ingredients:
- 4 salmon fillets (about 6 ounces each), skin-on or skinless
- Salt and pepper to taste
- 2 tablespoons olive oil
- 1/4 cup honey
- 2 tablespoons Dijon mustard
- 1 tablespoon whole grain mustard
- 2 cloves garlic, minced
- 1 tablespoon lemon juice
- Optional garnish: chopped fresh parsley or green onions

Instructions:

1. Season both sides of the salmon fillets with salt and pepper to taste.

2. In a small bowl, whisk together honey, Dijon mustard, whole grain mustard, minced garlic, and lemon juice to make the honey mustard glaze.

3. Heat olive oil in a large skillet over medium-high heat.

4. Place the salmon fillets in the skillet, skin-side down if they have skin. Cook for about 3-4 minutes until nicely seared and golden brown on the bottom.

5. Flip the salmon fillets and pour the honey mustard glaze over the top.

6. Reduce the heat to medium-low. Cover the skillet and let the salmon cook for another 5-6 minutes, or until the salmon is cooked to your desired level of doneness and the glaze has thickened slightly.

7. Spoon the glaze from the skillet over the salmon fillets occasionally while cooking.

8. Once the salmon is cooked, remove it from the skillet and set aside.

9. Optionally, you can boil the remaining glaze in the skillet for 1-2 minutes to further thicken it.

10. Serve the Honey Mustard Glazed Salmon hot, garnished with chopped fresh parsley or green onions if desired.

Enjoy your delicious and easy single-skillet Honey Mustard Glazed Salmon!

44. Thai Peanut Chicken Stir-Fry

Ingredients:

- 1 tablespoon vegetable oil
- 1 pound boneless, skinless chicken breasts, thinly sliced
- Salt and pepper to taste
- 1 red bell pepper, thinly sliced
- 1 yellow bell pepper, thinly sliced
- 1 cup broccoli florets
- 1 carrot, julienned or thinly sliced
- 2 cloves garlic, minced
- 1 tablespoon grated ginger
- 1/4 cup creamy peanut butter
- 2 tablespoons soy sauce
- 1 tablespoon rice vinegar
- 1 tablespoon honey or maple syrup
- 1 teaspoon sesame oil
- 1/4 cup chicken broth or water
- Crushed peanuts, for garnish
- Chopped cilantro, for garnish
- Cooked rice, for serving

Instructions:

1. Heat vegetable oil in a large skillet over medium-high heat.

2. Season the thinly sliced chicken breasts with salt and pepper. Add them to the skillet and cook for about 4-5 minutes until browned and cooked through. Remove the chicken from the skillet and set aside.

3. In the same skillet, add red bell pepper, yellow bell pepper, broccoli florets, and julienned carrot. Cook for about 4-5 minutes until the vegetables are tender-crisp.

4. Add minced garlic and grated ginger to the skillet. Cook for another minute until fragrant.

5. In a small bowl, whisk together creamy peanut butter, soy sauce, rice vinegar, honey or maple syrup, sesame oil, and chicken broth (or water) until smooth.

6. Pour the peanut sauce over the vegetables in the skillet. Stir well to combine.

7. Return the cooked chicken to the skillet, tossing everything together until the chicken and vegetables are coated with the sauce.

8. Let the stir-fry simmer for another 2-3 minutes to heat through and thicken the sauce slightly.

9. Serve the Thai Peanut Chicken Stir-Fry hot, over cooked rice. Garnish with crushed peanuts and chopped cilantro before serving.

Enjoy your delicious and easy single-skillet Thai Peanut Chicken Stir-Fry!

45. Brussels Sprouts and Bacon Skillet

Ingredients:

- 6 slices bacon, diced
- 1 pound Brussels sprouts, trimmed and halved
- Salt and pepper to taste
- 2 cloves garlic, minced
- 1/4 cup chicken broth or water
- 2 tablespoons balsamic vinegar
- 1 tablespoon honey or maple syrup
- Optional garnish: grated Parmesan cheese, chopped fresh parsley

Instructions:

1. Heat a large skillet over medium heat. Add the diced bacon and cook until crispy. Remove the cooked bacon from the skillet and set aside, leaving the bacon fat in the skillet.

2. In the same skillet with the bacon fat, add the halved Brussels sprouts in a single layer, cut side down. Season with salt and pepper to taste. Cook for about 5-7 minutes until the Brussels sprouts are browned and caramelized on the bottom.

3. Flip the Brussels sprouts and add minced garlic to the skillet. Cook for another 2-3 minutes until the garlic is fragrant.

4. Pour chicken broth (or water) into the skillet. Cover and let the Brussels sprouts steam for about 5-7 minutes, or until they are tender but still crisp.

5. Remove the lid and stir in balsamic vinegar and honey (or maple syrup) until the Brussels sprouts are evenly coated.

6. Return the cooked bacon to the skillet. Toss everything together until well combined.

7. Cook for another 1-2 minutes to heat through and allow the flavors to meld together.

8. Taste and adjust seasoning if needed.

9. Serve the Brussels Sprouts and Bacon Skillet hot, optionally garnished with grated Parmesan cheese and chopped fresh parsley.

Enjoy your delicious and easy single-skillet Brussels Sprouts and Bacon Skillet!

46. Cilantro Lime Shrimp

Ingredients:
- 1 pound large shrimp, peeled and deveined
- Salt and pepper to taste
- 2 tablespoons olive oil
- 3 cloves garlic, minced
- 1 teaspoon chili powder (optional)
- Juice of 2 limes
- Zest of 1 lime
- 1/4 cup chopped fresh cilantro
- Optional garnish: lime wedges, chopped fresh cilantro, sliced green onions

Instructions:
1. Pat the shrimp dry with paper towels and season them with salt, pepper, and chili powder (if using).

2. Heat olive oil in a large skillet over medium-high heat.

3. Add minced garlic to the skillet and cook for about 1 minute until fragrant.

4. Add the seasoned shrimp to the skillet in a single layer. Cook for about 2-3 minutes on each side until pink and opaque.

5. Reduce the heat to low. Add lime juice and lime zest to the skillet, stirring to combine.

6. Stir in chopped fresh cilantro, reserving some for garnish if desired.

7. Let the shrimp simmer in the lime and cilantro mixture for another minute or two, allowing the flavors to meld together.

8. Taste and adjust seasoning if needed.

9. Serve the Cilantro Lime Shrimp hot, garnished with additional chopped cilantro and lime wedges if desired.

Enjoy your delicious and easy single-skillet Cilantro Lime Shrimp!

47. One-Pot Chicken Alfredo

Ingredients:
- 2 boneless, skinless chicken breasts, cut into bite-sized pieces
- Salt and pepper to taste
- 2 tablespoons olive oil
- 3 cloves garlic, minced
- 2 cups chicken broth
- 1 cup heavy cream
- 8 ounces fettuccine pasta
- 1 cup grated Parmesan cheese
- 1 tablespoon chopped fresh parsley (optional)

Instructions:

1. Season the chicken breast pieces with salt and pepper to taste.

2. Heat olive oil in a large skillet over medium-high heat.

3. Add the seasoned chicken breast pieces to the skillet. Cook for about 5-6 minutes until golden brown and cooked through. Remove the chicken from the skillet and set aside.

4. In the same skillet, add minced garlic and cook for about 1 minute until fragrant.

5. Pour chicken broth and heavy cream into the skillet, stirring to combine.

6. Break the fettuccine pasta in half and add it to the skillet, ensuring it's submerged in the liquid.

7. Bring the mixture to a simmer. Reduce the heat to medium-low and let it cook, stirring occasionally, for about 12-15 minutes until the pasta is cooked and the sauce has thickened.

8. Once the pasta is cooked, stir in grated Parmesan cheese until melted and incorporated into the sauce.

9. Return the cooked chicken to the skillet, stirring to combine with the pasta and sauce.

10. Let the chicken Alfredo simmer for another 2-3 minutes to heat through.

11. Taste and adjust seasoning if needed.

12. Serve the One-Pot Chicken Alfredo hot, optionally garnished with chopped fresh parsley.

Enjoy your delicious and easy single-skillet One-Pot Chicken Alfredo!

48. Soy Ginger Glazed Cod

Ingredients:
- 4 cod fillets (about 6 ounces each)
- Salt and pepper to taste
- 2 tablespoons olive oil
- 3 tablespoons soy sauce
- 2 tablespoons honey
- 1 tablespoon rice vinegar
- 1 tablespoon grated ginger
- 2 cloves garlic, minced
- 1 tablespoon cornstarch
- 2 tablespoons water
- Optional garnish: sesame seeds, sliced green onions

Instructions:

1. Season both sides of the cod fillets with salt and pepper to taste.

2. In a small bowl, whisk together soy sauce, honey, rice vinegar, grated ginger, and minced garlic to make the glaze.

3. In a separate small bowl, mix cornstarch with water to make a slurry.

4. Heat olive oil in a large skillet over medium-high heat.

5. Place the cod fillets in the skillet and cook for about 3-4 minutes on each side until lightly browned and cooked through.

6. Reduce the heat to low. Pour the soy ginger glaze over the cod fillets in the skillet.

7. Pour the cornstarch slurry into the skillet, stirring gently to combine with the glaze. Allow the glaze to thicken slightly.

8. Spoon the glaze over the cod fillets to coat them evenly.

9. Cook for another 1-2 minutes, until the glaze is thickened and the cod fillets are fully coated.

10. Remove from heat and transfer the glazed cod fillets to serving plates.

11. Optionally, garnish with sesame seeds and sliced green onions before serving.

12. Serve the Soy Ginger Glazed Cod hot, with your choice of side dishes like rice or vegetables

49. Vegetarian Taco Skillet

Ingredients:

- 1 tablespoon olive oil
- 1 onion, diced
- 1 bell pepper, diced (any color)
- 1 zucchini, diced
- 1 cup corn kernels (fresh, frozen, or canned)
- 1 can (15 ounces) black beans, drained and rinsed
- 1 can (14.5 ounces) diced tomatoes, undrained
- 1 packet (1 ounce) taco seasoning
- Salt and pepper to taste
- 1 cup shredded cheese (cheddar, Monterey Jack, or Mexican blend)
- Optional toppings: diced avocado, chopped cilantro, sour cream, salsa, lime wedges, tortilla chips

Instructions:

1. Heat olive oil in a large skillet over medium heat.

2. Add diced onion and diced bell pepper to the skillet. Cook for about 3-4 minutes until softened.

3. Stir in diced zucchini and corn kernels. Cook for another 2-3 minutes until the vegetables are tender-crisp.

4. Add drained and rinsed black beans, diced tomatoes (with their juices), and taco seasoning to the skillet. Stir well to combine.

5. Season with salt and pepper to taste. Cook for another 2-3 minutes to heat everything through and allow the flavors to meld together.

6. Sprinkle shredded cheese evenly over the top of the skillet mixture.

7. Cover the skillet and let it simmer for about 2-3 minutes until the cheese is melted and bubbly.

8. Remove the skillet from heat.

9. Optionally, garnish with diced avocado, chopped cilantro, sour cream, salsa, and lime wedges.

10. Serve the Vegetarian Taco Skillet hot, optionally with tortilla chips for scooping.

50. Sausage and Potato Hash

Ingredients:
- 1 tablespoon olive oil
- 1 pound sausage (such as breakfast sausage or Italian sausage), casings removed if necessary
- 1 onion, diced
- 2 cloves garlic, minced
- 1 bell pepper, diced (any color)
- 1 pound potatoes, diced into small cubes
- 1 teaspoon paprika
- Salt and pepper to taste
- Optional toppings: chopped fresh parsley, grated cheese, hot sauce

Instructions:

1. Heat olive oil in a large skillet over medium heat.

2. Add sausage to the skillet, breaking it up with a spatula. Cook for about 5-6 minutes until browned and cooked through.

3. Add diced onion to the skillet and cook for another 2-3 minutes until softened.

4. Stir in minced garlic and diced bell pepper. Cook for another 2-3 minutes until the bell pepper is tender.

5. Add diced potatoes to the skillet. Season with paprika, salt, and pepper to taste. Stir well to combine all ingredients.

6. Spread the mixture evenly in the skillet. Let it cook without stirring for about 5 minutes to allow the potatoes to brown on the bottom.

7. Stir the mixture and spread it out again. Let it cook for another 5-7 minutes until the potatoes are cooked through and crispy on the outside.

8. Taste and adjust seasoning if needed.

9. Optionally, top the Sausage and Potato Hash with chopped fresh parsley, grated cheese, or hot sauce before serving.

10. Serve the hash hot, straight from the skillet.

Enjoy your delicious and easy single-skillet Sausage and Potato Hash!

51. Mushroom Stroganoff

Ingredients:
- 8 ounces egg noodles or any pasta of your choice
- 2 tablespoons butter
- 1 onion, diced
- 3 cloves garlic, minced
- 1 pound mushrooms (such as button or cremini), sliced
- 2 tablespoons all-purpose flour
- 2 cups vegetable broth or mushroom broth
- 1 tablespoon soy sauce
- 1 teaspoon Dijon mustard
- 1/2 cup sour cream
- Salt and pepper to taste
- Chopped fresh parsley, for garnish (optional)

Instructions:

1. Cook the egg noodles or pasta according to the package instructions until al dente. Drain and set aside.

2. In the same skillet, melt the butter over medium heat.

3. Add the diced onion to the skillet and cook for about 3-4 minutes until softened.

4. Stir in the minced garlic and sliced mushrooms. Cook for another 5-6 minutes until the mushrooms are tender and browned.

5. Sprinkle the flour over the mushrooms and stir to combine. Cook for 1-2 minutes to cook off the raw flour taste.

6. Gradually pour in the vegetable broth or mushroom broth, stirring constantly to prevent lumps from forming.

7. Stir in the soy sauce and Dijon mustard. Bring the mixture to a simmer and let it cook for about 5-7 minutes until slightly thickened.

8. Reduce the heat to low. Stir in the sour cream until smooth and well combined.

9. Season the mushroom stroganoff with salt and pepper to taste.

10. Add the cooked egg noodles or pasta to the skillet. Stir until the noodles are coated with the creamy mushroom sauce.

11. Let the mushroom stroganoff simmer for another 2-3 minutes to heat through.

12. Optionally, garnish with chopped fresh parsley before serving.

13. Serve the Mushroom Stroganoff hot, straight from the skillet

52. Skillet Ratatouille Pasta

Ingredients:
- 8 ounces penne pasta
- 2 tablespoons olive oil
- 1 onion, diced
- 2 cloves garlic, minced
- 1 eggplant, diced
- 1 zucchini, diced
- 1 yellow bell pepper, diced
- 1 red bell pepper, diced
- 1 can (14.5 ounces) diced tomatoes, undrained
- 1 teaspoon dried basil
- 1 teaspoon dried oregano
- Salt and pepper to taste
- Grated Parmesan cheese, for serving
- Chopped fresh basil, for garnish (optional)

Instructions:

1. Cook the penne pasta according to the package instructions until al dente. Drain and set aside.

2. In the same skillet, heat olive oil over medium heat.

3. Add diced onion and minced garlic to the skillet. Cook for about 2-3 minutes until softened and fragrant.

4. Add diced eggplant, diced zucchini, diced yellow bell pepper, and diced red bell pepper to the skillet. Cook for about 5-7 minutes until the vegetables are tender.

5. Stir in diced tomatoes (with their juices), dried basil, and dried oregano. Season with salt and pepper to taste. Cook for another 5 minutes to allow the flavors to meld together.

6. Add the cooked penne pasta to the skillet. Stir well to combine with the ratatouille mixture.

7. Let the skillet ratatouille pasta simmer for another 2-3 minutes to heat through.

8. Taste and adjust seasoning if needed.

9. Serve the Skillet Ratatouille Pasta hot, sprinkled with grated Parmesan cheese and garnished with chopped fresh basil if desired.

53. Honey Sriracha Chicken and Broccoli

Ingredients:

- 1 pound boneless, skinless chicken breasts, cut into bite-sized pieces
- Salt and pepper to taste
- 1 tablespoon olive oil
- 2 cups broccoli florets
- 3 cloves garlic, minced
- 1/4 cup honey
- 2 tablespoons soy sauce
- 1 tablespoon sriracha sauce (adjust to taste)
- 1 tablespoon rice vinegar
- Sesame seeds, for garnish (optional)
- Sliced green onions, for garnish (optional)

Instructions:

1. Season the chicken breast pieces with salt and pepper to taste.

2. Heat olive oil in a large skillet over medium-high heat.

3. Add the seasoned chicken breast pieces to the skillet. Cook for about 5-6 minutes until browned and cooked through.

4. Remove the cooked chicken from the skillet and set aside.

5. In the same skillet, add broccoli florets and minced garlic. Cook for about 3-4 minutes until the broccoli is tender-crisp.

6. While the broccoli is cooking, in a small bowl, whisk together honey, soy sauce, sriracha sauce, and rice vinegar to make the sauce.

7. Return the cooked chicken to the skillet with the broccoli.

8. Pour the honey sriracha sauce over the chicken and broccoli in the skillet. Stir well to coat everything evenly.

9. Let the skillet simmer for another 2-3 minutes, allowing the sauce to thicken slightly and the flavors to meld together.

10. Taste and adjust seasoning if needed.

11. Optionally, garnish with sesame seeds and sliced green onions before serving. Serve the Honey Sriracha Chicken and Broccoli hot, over cooked rice or noodles.

54. Creamy Garlic Parmesan Orzo

Ingredients:
- 1 cup orzo pasta
- 2 tablespoons butter
- 3 cloves garlic, minced
- 2 cups chicken broth or vegetable broth
- 1 cup heavy cream
- 1/2 cup grated Parmesan cheese
- Salt and pepper to taste
- Chopped fresh parsley, for garnish (optional)

Instructions:

1. In a large skillet, melt the butter over medium heat.

2. Add minced garlic to the skillet and cook for about 1 minute until fragrant.

3. Pour in the chicken broth (or vegetable broth) and bring it to a boil.

4. Add the orzo pasta to the skillet. Stir well to combine with the broth.

5. Reduce the heat to low and let the orzo simmer, covered, for about 10-12 minutes, or until the orzo is cooked through and most of the liquid is absorbed.

6. Stir in the heavy cream and grated Parmesan cheese until smooth and creamy.

7. Let the creamy garlic Parmesan orzo simmer for another 2-3 minutes to thicken the sauce.

8. Season with salt and pepper to taste.

9. Optionally, garnish with chopped fresh parsley before serving.

10. Serve the Creamy Garlic Parmesan Orzo hot, as a side dish or as a main course.

Enjoy your delicious and easy single-skillet Creamy Garlic Parmesan Orzo!

55. Shrimp and Broccoli Stir-Fry

Ingredients:

- 1 pound large shrimp, peeled and deveined
- Salt and pepper to taste
- 2 tablespoons vegetable oil
- 3 cups broccoli florets
- 3 cloves garlic, minced
- 1 tablespoon grated ginger
- 1/4 cup soy sauce
- 2 tablespoons oyster sauce
- 1 tablespoon honey or brown sugar
- 1 tablespoon cornstarch
- 1/4 cup water
- Optional garnish: sliced green onions, sesame seeds

Instructions:

1. Season the shrimp with salt and pepper to taste.

2. In a small bowl, mix soy sauce, oyster sauce, honey (or brown sugar), cornstarch, and water. Set aside.

3. Heat vegetable oil in a large skillet over medium-high heat.

4. Add shrimp to the skillet and cook for about 2 minutes on each side until pink and opaque. Remove the shrimp from the skillet and set aside.

5. In the same skillet, add broccoli florets. Cook for about 3-4 minutes until tender-crisp.

6. Add minced garlic and grated ginger to the skillet. Cook for another 1-2 minutes until fragrant.

7. Return the cooked shrimp to the skillet with the broccoli.

8. Pour the sauce mixture over the shrimp and broccoli in the skillet. Stir well to coat everything evenly.

9. Let the stir-fry simmer for another 2-3 minutes until the sauce thickens and coats the shrimp and broccoli.

10. Taste and adjust seasoning if needed. Optionally, garnish with sliced green onions and sesame seeds before serving. Serve the Shrimp and Broccoli Stir-Fry hot, over cooked rice or noodles.

56. Butternut Squash and Kale Pasta

Ingredients:
- 8 ounces pasta (such as penne, fusilli, or farfalle)
- 2 tablespoons olive oil
- 1 small butternut squash, peeled, seeded, and diced
- Salt and pepper to taste
- 2 cloves garlic, minced
- 4 cups chopped kale leaves, stems removed
- 1/4 teaspoon red pepper flakes (optional)
- 1/4 cup vegetable broth or water
- 1/4 cup grated Parmesan cheese, plus extra for serving
- Optional garnish: chopped fresh parsley, toasted pine nuts

Instructions:

1. Cook the pasta according to the package instructions until al dente. Drain and set aside.

2. In the same skillet, heat olive oil over medium heat.

3. Add diced butternut squash to the skillet. Season with salt and pepper to taste. Cook for about 8-10 minutes until the squash is tender and lightly browned.

4. Add minced garlic and red pepper flakes (if using) to the skillet. Cook for another 1-2 minutes until fragrant.

5. Stir in chopped kale leaves and vegetable broth (or water) to the skillet. Cover and cook for about 5 minutes until the kale is wilted and tender.

6. Return the cooked pasta to the skillet. Stir well to combine with the butternut squash and kale mixture.

7. Add grated Parmesan cheese to the skillet. Toss everything together until the cheese is melted and incorporated.

8. Taste and adjust seasoning if needed.

9. Optionally, garnish with chopped fresh parsley, toasted pine nuts, and extra grated Parmesan cheese before serving.

10. Serve the Butternut Squash and Kale Pasta hot.

Enjoy your delicious and easy single-skillet Butternut Squash and Kale Pasta!

57. Cajun Chicken Pasta

Ingredients:

- 8 ounces penne pasta
- 2 boneless, skinless chicken breasts, cut into bite-sized pieces
- 2 tablespoons Cajun seasoning
- Salt and pepper to taste
- 2 tablespoons olive oil
- 2 cloves garlic, minced
- 1 bell pepper, thinly sliced
- 1 small onion, thinly sliced
- 1 cup cherry tomatoes, halved
- 1 cup heavy cream
- 1/2 cup chicken broth
- 1/4 cup grated Parmesan cheese
- Chopped fresh parsley, for garnish (optional)

Instructions:

1. Cook the penne pasta according to the package instructions until al dente. Drain and set aside.

2. In a small bowl, toss the chicken breast pieces with Cajun seasoning, salt, and pepper until evenly coated.

3. Heat olive oil in a large skillet over medium-high heat.

4. Add the seasoned chicken breast pieces to the skillet. Cook for about 5-6 minutes until browned and cooked through. Remove the chicken from the skillet and set aside.

5. In the same skillet, add minced garlic, thinly sliced bell pepper, and thinly sliced onion. Cook for about 3-4 minutes until the vegetables are tender.

6. Stir in halved cherry tomatoes and cook for another 2 minutes until softened.

7. Pour in heavy cream and chicken broth. Bring the mixture to a simmer.

8. Return the cooked chicken to the skillet. Stir well to combine with the sauce.

9. Sprinkle grated Parmesan cheese over the skillet. Stir until the cheese is melted and the sauce is creamy.

10. Add the cooked penne pasta to the skillet. Toss everything together until the pasta is coated with the creamy Cajun sauce.

11. Let the Cajun Chicken Pasta simmer for another 2-3 minutes to heat through. Taste and adjust seasoning if needed.

12. Optionally, garnish with chopped fresh parsley before serving. Serve the Cajun Chicken Pasta hot.

58. Teriyaki Beef and Vegetable Stir-Fry

Ingredients:
- 1 pound flank steak, thinly sliced against the grain
- 1/4 cup soy sauce
- 2 tablespoons honey
- 2 tablespoons rice vinegar
- 1 tablespoon sesame oil
- 2 cloves garlic, minced
- 1 teaspoon grated ginger
- 2 tablespoons vegetable oil
- 1 onion, thinly sliced
- 2 bell peppers, thinly sliced (any color)
- 2 cups broccoli florets
- Salt and pepper to taste
- Sesame seeds, for garnish (optional)
- Sliced green onions, for garnish (optional)

Instructions:

1. In a small bowl, whisk together soy sauce, honey, rice vinegar, sesame oil, minced garlic, and grated ginger to make the teriyaki sauce. Set aside.

2. Heat vegetable oil in a large skillet over medium-high heat.

3. Add thinly sliced flank steak to the skillet. Cook for about 2-3 minutes until browned.

4. Remove the beef from the skillet and set aside.

5. In the same skillet, add sliced onion and cook for about 2 minutes until softened.

6. Add thinly sliced bell peppers and broccoli florets to the skillet. Cook for another 3-4 minutes until the vegetables are tender-crisp.

7. Return the cooked beef to the skillet with the vegetables.

8. Pour the teriyaki sauce over the beef and vegetables in the skillet. Stir well to coat everything evenly.

9. Let the stir-fry simmer for another 2-3 minutes until the sauce thickens slightly.

10. Taste and adjust seasoning with salt and pepper if needed.

11. Optionally, garnish with sesame seeds and sliced green onions before serving.

12. Serve the Teriyaki Beef and Vegetable Stir-Fry hot, over cooked rice or noodles.

59. Caprese Quinoa

Ingredients:
- 1 cup quinoa, rinsed and drained
- 2 cups water or vegetable broth
- 1 tablespoon olive oil
- 2 cloves garlic, minced
- 1 pint cherry tomatoes, halved
- 8 ounces fresh mozzarella, diced
- 1/4 cup fresh basil leaves, chopped
- Salt and pepper to taste
- Balsamic glaze, for drizzling (optional)

Instructions:

1. In a large skillet, heat olive oil over medium heat.

2. Add minced garlic to the skillet and cook for about 1 minute until fragrant.

3. Add rinsed and drained quinoa to the skillet. Stir and toast the quinoa for about 2 minutes.

4. Pour water or vegetable broth into the skillet. Bring to a boil.

5. Once boiling, reduce heat to low, cover, and let the quinoa simmer for about 15-20 minutes, or until all liquid is absorbed and quinoa is tender.

6. Once the quinoa is cooked, fluff it with a fork.

7. Add halved cherry tomatoes, diced fresh mozzarella, and chopped basil to the skillet with the cooked quinoa.

8. Season with salt and pepper to taste. Stir well to combine all ingredients.

9. Let the mixture cook for another 2-3 minutes until the cheese starts to melt and the tomatoes soften slightly.

10. Optionally, drizzle with balsamic glaze before serving.

11. Serve the Caprese Quinoa hot as a main dish or side dish.

Enjoy your delicious and easy single-skillet Caprese Quinoa!

60. Skillet Cornbread

Ingredients:
- 1 cup cornmeal
- 1 cup all-purpose flour
- 1/4 cup granulated sugar
- 1 tablespoon baking powder
- 1/2 teaspoon baking soda
- 1/2 teaspoon salt
- 1 cup buttermilk
- 1/2 cup unsalted butter, melted
- 2 large eggs
- 1 cup corn kernels (fresh, frozen, or canned)
- Optional add-ins: diced jalapenos, shredded cheese, chopped green onions

Instructions:

1. Preheat your oven to 375°F (190°C). Place a 10-inch cast iron skillet in the oven to heat while you prepare the batter.

2. In a large mixing bowl, whisk together the cornmeal, flour, sugar, baking powder, baking soda, and salt.

3. In a separate bowl, mix together the buttermilk, melted butter, and eggs until well combined.

4. Pour the wet ingredients into the dry ingredients and stir until just combined. Be careful not to overmix.

5. Fold in the corn kernels (and any optional add-ins, if using).

6. Carefully remove the hot skillet from the oven using oven mitts. Coat the skillet with a thin layer of butter or oil to prevent sticking.

7. Pour the cornbread batter into the hot skillet and spread it evenly.

8. Bake in the preheated oven for 20-25 minutes, or until the cornbread is golden brown on top and a toothpick inserted into the center comes out clean.

9. Remove the skillet from the oven and let the cornbread cool for a few minutes before slicing and serving.

10. Serve the skillet cornbread warm as a side dish or as part of a meal

61. Lemon Herb Tilapia

Ingredients:
- 4 tilapia fillets
- Salt and pepper to taste
- 2 tablespoons olive oil
- 2 cloves garlic, minced
- Zest and juice of 1 lemon
- 1 teaspoon dried thyme
- 1 teaspoon dried parsley
- 1/2 teaspoon dried oregano
- 1/4 teaspoon paprika
- Lemon slices, for garnish
- Chopped fresh parsley, for garnish

Instructions:
1. Pat dry the tilapia fillets with paper towels and season both sides with salt and pepper.

2. In a small bowl, mix together the minced garlic, lemon zest, lemon juice, dried thyme, dried parsley, dried oregano, and paprika to make the herb mixture.

3. Heat olive oil in a large skillet over medium-high heat.

4. Place the seasoned tilapia fillets in the skillet and cook for about 3-4 minutes on each side, or until the fish is cooked through and easily flakes with a fork.

5. Reduce the heat to low and add the herb mixture to the skillet. Spoon the mixture over the tilapia fillets, ensuring they are evenly coated.

6. Let the fish cook for another 1-2 minutes, allowing the flavors to meld together.

7. Garnish the Lemon Herb Tilapia with lemon slices and chopped fresh parsley before serving.

8. Serve the Lemon Herb Tilapia hot, with your choice of side dishes like rice or vegetables.

Enjoy your delicious and easy single-skillet Lemon Herb Tilapia!

62. Sesame Ginger Tofu Stir-Fry

Ingredients:

- 14 ounces extra-firm tofu, drained and pressed
- 2 tablespoons soy sauce
- 1 tablespoon rice vinegar
- 1 tablespoon sesame oil
- 1 tablespoon honey or maple syrup
- 1 tablespoon cornstarch
- 2 cloves garlic, minced
- 2 tablespoons vegetable oil
- 1 tablespoon grated ginger
- 1 bell pepper, thinly sliced
- 1 cup broccoli florets
- 1 carrot, thinly sliced
- 2 green onions, chopped (for garnish)
- Sesame seeds (for garnish)

Instructions:

1. Cut the pressed tofu into cubes.

2. In a small bowl, mix together soy sauce, rice vinegar, sesame oil, honey (or maple syrup), and cornstarch to make the sauce. Set aside.

3. Heat vegetable oil in a large skillet over medium-high heat.

4. Add the tofu cubes to the skillet. Cook for about 5-7 minutes, flipping occasionally, until they are golden brown and crispy on all sides. Remove the tofu from the skillet and set aside.

5. In the same skillet, add minced garlic and grated ginger. Cook for about 1 minute until fragrant.

6. Add thinly sliced bell pepper, broccoli florets, and thinly sliced carrot to the skillet. Stir-fry for about 5-7 minutes until the vegetables are tender-crisp.

7. Return the cooked tofu to the skillet with the vegetables.

8. Pour the sauce over the tofu and vegetables. Stir well to coat everything evenly.

9. Let the stir-fry simmer for another 2-3 minutes, allowing the sauce to thicken.

10. Taste and adjust seasoning if needed.

11. Garnish the Sesame Ginger Tofu Stir-Fry with chopped green onions and sesame seeds.

12. Serve the stir-fry hot, over cooked rice or noodles.

Enjoy your delicious and easy single-skillet Sesame Ginger Tofu Stir-Fry!

63. Creamy Spinach and Mushroom Gnocchi

Ingredients:

- 16 ounces gnocchi
- 2 tablespoons butter
- 8 ounces mushrooms, sliced
- 3 cloves garlic, minced
- 4 cups fresh spinach leaves
- 1 cup heavy cream
- 1/2 cup grated Parmesan cheese
- Salt and pepper to taste
- Optional: Red pepper flakes, for a spicy kick
- Chopped fresh parsley, for garnish

Instructions:

1. Cook the gnocchi according to the package instructions. Drain and set aside.

2. In a large skillet, melt the butter over medium heat.

3. Add the sliced mushrooms to the skillet. Cook for about 5-7 minutes until they are golden brown and tender.

4. Add the minced garlic to the skillet and cook for another 1-2 minutes until fragrant.

5. Stir in the fresh spinach leaves. Cook for a few minutes until wilted.

6. Pour in the heavy cream and stir well to combine with the mushroom and spinach mixture.

7. Add the cooked gnocchi to the skillet. Stir gently to coat the gnocchi with the creamy sauce.

8. Sprinkle grated Parmesan cheese over the skillet. Stir until the cheese is melted and the sauce is creamy.

9. Season with salt and pepper to taste. Add red pepper flakes for a spicy kick if desired.

10. Let the creamy spinach and mushroom gnocchi simmer for a few minutes until heated through.

11. Garnish with chopped fresh parsley before serving. Serve the creamy spinach and mushroom gnocchi hot.Enjoy your delicious and easy single-skillet Creamy Spinach and Mushroom Gnocchi!

64. One-Pan Balsamic Chicken and Vegetables

Ingredients:

- 4 boneless, skinless chicken breasts
- Salt and pepper to taste
- 2 tablespoons olive oil
- 1 red bell pepper, sliced
- 1 yellow bell pepper, sliced
- 1 zucchini, sliced
- 1 yellow squash, sliced
- 1 onion, sliced
- 4 cloves garlic, minced
- 1/4 cup balsamic vinegar
- 2 tablespoons honey
- 1 teaspoon dried thyme
- 1 teaspoon dried rosemary
- Chopped fresh parsley, for garnish

Instructions:

1. Season the chicken breasts with salt and pepper to taste.

2. In a large skillet, heat olive oil over medium-high heat.

3. Add the seasoned chicken breasts to the skillet. Cook for about 5-6 minutes on each side, or until browned and cooked through. Remove the chicken from the skillet and set aside.

4. In the same skillet, add sliced red bell pepper, yellow bell pepper, zucchini, yellow squash, onion, and minced garlic. Cook for about 5-6 minutes until the vegetables are tender-crisp.

5. In a small bowl, whisk together balsamic vinegar, honey, dried thyme, and dried rosemary.

6. Pour the balsamic mixture over the vegetables in the skillet. Stir well to coat the vegetables evenly.

7. Return the cooked chicken breasts to the skillet, nestling them among the vegetables.

8. Let the chicken and vegetables simmer in the balsamic sauce for another 2-3 minutes to heat through and absorb the flavors.

9. Taste and adjust seasoning if needed.

10. Garnish with chopped fresh parsley before serving.

11. Serve the One-Pan Balsamic Chicken and Vegetables hot.

65. Sweet and Sour Tofu

Ingredients:

- 14 ounces extra-firm tofu, drained and pressed
- 2 tablespoons cornstarch
- 2 tablespoons vegetable oil
- 1 bell pepper, diced
- 1 onion, diced
- 1 cup pineapple chunks (fresh or canned)
- 1/4 cup ketchup
- 2 tablespoons brown sugar
- 1 tablespoon cornstarch mixed with 2 tablespoons water (for thickening)
- Salt and pepper to taste
- 3 tablespoons rice vinegar
- 2 tablespoons soy sauce
- Cooked rice, for serving
- Optional garnish: chopped green onions, sesame seeds

Instructions:

1. Cut the pressed tofu into cubes and toss them with 2 tablespoons of cornstarch until coated.

2. Heat vegetable oil in a large skillet over medium-high heat.

3. Add the coated tofu cubes to the skillet and cook for about 5-7 minutes, flipping occasionally, until they are golden brown and crispy on all sides. Remove the tofu from the skillet and set aside.

4. In the same skillet, add diced bell pepper and onion. Cook for about 3-4 minutes until they are tender.

5. Add pineapple chunks to the skillet and cook for another 1-2 minutes until heated through.

6. In a small bowl, whisk together ketchup, rice vinegar, soy sauce, brown sugar, and cornstarch-water mixture.

7. Pour the sauce mixture into the skillet with the vegetables. Stir well to combine.

8. Return the cooked tofu to the skillet and toss everything together until the tofu is coated with the sweet and sour sauce.

9. Let the mixture simmer for another 2-3 minutes until the sauce thickens. Taste and adjust seasoning with salt and pepper if needed.

10. Serve the Sweet and Sour Tofu hot over cooked rice. Optionally, garnish with chopped green onions and sesame seeds before serving.

66. Skillet Chicken and Rice

Ingredients:

- 1 tablespoon olive oil
- 4 boneless, skinless chicken breasts
- Salt and pepper to taste
- 1 onion, diced
- 2 cloves garlic, minced
- 1 bell pepper, diced
- 1 cup long-grain white rice
- 2 cups chicken broth
- 1 teaspoon dried thyme
- 1 teaspoon paprika
- 1/2 teaspoon garlic powder
- 1/2 teaspoon onion powder
- 1/4 teaspoon cayenne pepper (optional)
- Chopped fresh parsley, for garnish (optional)

Instructions:

1. Heat olive oil in a large skillet over medium-high heat.

2. Season the chicken breasts with salt and pepper to taste.

3. Place the chicken breasts in the skillet and cook for about 5-6 minutes on each side, or until browned and cooked through. Remove the chicken from the skillet and set aside.

4. In the same skillet, add diced onion, minced garlic, and diced bell pepper. Cook for about 3-4 minutes until the vegetables are softened.

5. Stir in the rice and cook for another 1-2 minutes until lightly toasted.

6. Pour in the chicken broth and add dried thyme, paprika, garlic powder, onion powder, and cayenne pepper (if using). Stir well to combine.

7. Return the cooked chicken breasts to the skillet, nestling them into the rice mixture.

8. Bring the mixture to a simmer, then reduce the heat to low. Cover and let it simmer for about 18-20 minutes, or until the rice is cooked and most of the liquid is absorbed.

9. Check for doneness of the rice and chicken. If needed, let it cook for a few more minutes until fully cooked.

10. Once everything is cooked through, remove the skillet from the heat. Garnish with chopped fresh parsley before serving, if desired. Serve the Skillet Chicken and Rice hot.

67. Vegetarian Fajita Skillet

Ingredients:

- 2 tablespoons olive oil
- 1 onion, thinly sliced
- 1 red bell pepper, thinly sliced
- 1 green bell pepper, thinly sliced
- 1 yellow bell pepper, thinly sliced
- 1 teaspoon chili powder
- 1 teaspoon ground cumin
- 1/2 teaspoon smoked paprika
- 1/2 teaspoon garlic powder
- Salt and pepper to taste
- 1 (15 oz) can black beans, drained and rinsed
- 1 cup corn kernels (fresh, frozen, or canned)
- Juice of 1 lime
- 1/4 cup chopped fresh cilantro
- Tortillas, for serving
- Optional toppings: diced avocado, shredded cheese, salsa, sour cream, lime wedges

Instructions:

1. Heat olive oil in a large skillet over medium-high heat.

2. Add thinly sliced onion and bell peppers to the skillet. Cook for about 5-7 minutes, stirring occasionally, until the vegetables are softened and slightly charred.

3. Sprinkle chili powder, cumin, smoked paprika, garlic powder, salt, and pepper over the vegetables. Stir well to coat evenly.

4. Add drained black beans and corn kernels to the skillet. Cook for another 2-3 minutes until heated through.

5. Squeeze lime juice over the skillet and sprinkle chopped fresh cilantro on top. Stir to combine.

6. Taste and adjust seasoning if needed.

7. Serve the Vegetarian Fajita Skillet hot with tortillas and optional toppings such as diced avocado, shredded cheese, salsa, sour cream, and lime wedges.

68. Sausage and Potato Skillet

Ingredients:

- 1 lb (450g) sausage (any type you prefer, such as Italian sausage or breakfast sausage), sliced
- 1 lb (450g) baby potatoes, halved or quartered
- 1 onion, chopped
- 2 cloves garlic, minced
- 1 bell pepper, chopped (any color)
- 1 teaspoon dried thyme
- 1 teaspoon dried rosemary
- Salt and pepper to taste
- 2 tablespoons olive oil
- Chopped fresh parsley for garnish (optional)

Instructions:

1. Heat olive oil in a large skillet over medium heat.

2. Add the sliced sausage to the skillet. Cook, stirring occasionally, until the sausage is browned and cooked through, about 5-7 minutes.

3. Remove the cooked sausage from the skillet and set aside.

4. In the same skillet, add the halved baby potatoes. Cook for about 10 minutes, stirring occasionally, until they start to brown and soften.

5. Add the chopped onion, minced garlic, and chopped bell pepper to the skillet with the potatoes. Cook for another 5 minutes until the vegetables are tender.

6. Return the cooked sausage to the skillet with the potatoes and vegetables.

7. Sprinkle dried thyme, dried rosemary, salt, and pepper over the skillet. Stir well to combine all ingredients.

8. Cook for another 2-3 minutes until everything is heated through and the flavors are melded together.

9. Taste and adjust seasoning if needed.

10. Garnish with chopped fresh parsley before serving, if desired.

11. Serve the Sausage and Potato Skillet hot as a delicious and hearty meal.

69. One-Pot Lemon Garlic Shrimp Pasta

Ingredients:
- 8 oz (225g) spaghetti or linguine pasta
- 1 lb (450g) shrimp, peeled and deveined
- 4 cloves garlic, minced
- 2 tablespoons olive oil
- 3 cups chicken broth
- 1 lemon, zest and juice
- 1/4 teaspoon red pepper flakes (optional)
- Salt and pepper to taste
- 1/4 cup grated Parmesan cheese
- 2 tablespoons chopped fresh parsley, for garnish

Instructions:

1. In a large skillet, heat olive oil over medium heat. Add minced garlic and cook for about 1 minute until fragrant.

2. Add chicken broth to the skillet and bring it to a boil.

3. Break the spaghetti or linguine pasta in half and add it to the skillet. Stir well to submerge the pasta in the broth.

4. Cook the pasta according to the package instructions, stirring occasionally, until al dente and most of the broth is absorbed, about 8-10 minutes.

5. Once the pasta is cooked, add the shrimp to the skillet. Cook for about 3-4 minutes until the shrimp turn pink and opaque.

6. Stir in lemon zest, lemon juice, red pepper flakes (if using), salt, and pepper.

7. Sprinkle grated Parmesan cheese over the skillet and stir until the cheese is melted and the sauce is creamy.

8. Taste and adjust seasoning if needed.

9. Remove the skillet from the heat and garnish with chopped fresh parsley.

10. Serve the One-Pot Lemon Garlic Shrimp Pasta hot.

Enjoy your delicious and easy single-skillet One-Pot Lemon Garlic Shrimp Pasta!

70. Broccoli and Cheddar Stuffed Chicken

Ingredients:
- 4 boneless, skinless chicken breasts
- Salt and pepper to taste
- 1 cup broccoli florets, finely chopped
- 1 cup shredded cheddar cheese
- 2 tablespoons olive oil
- 2 cloves garlic, minced
- 1/2 cup chicken broth
- 1/2 cup heavy cream
- 1 tablespoon Dijon mustard
- 1 tablespoon chopped fresh parsley (optional, for garnish)

Instructions:

1. Preheat your oven to 375°F (190°C).

2. Using a sharp knife, make a horizontal slit along the side of each chicken breast to form a pocket. Be careful not to cut all the way through.

3. Season the inside of each chicken breast pocket with salt and pepper.

4. In a small bowl, mix together chopped broccoli florets and shredded cheddar cheese.

5. Stuff each chicken breast with the broccoli and cheddar mixture, dividing it evenly among the chicken breasts.

6. In a large skillet, heat olive oil over medium-high heat.

7. Add minced garlic to the skillet and cook for about 1 minute until fragrant.

8. Place the stuffed chicken breasts in the skillet and cook for about 3-4 minutes on each side until golden brown.

9. Remove the skillet from the heat and pour chicken broth and heavy cream into the skillet.

10. Add Dijon mustard to the skillet and stir well to combine with the broth and cream.

11. Transfer the skillet to the preheated oven and bake for about 20-25 minutes, or until the chicken is cooked through and the internal temperature reaches 165°F (74°C).

12. Once cooked, remove the skillet from the oven and let the chicken rest for a few minutes.

13. Garnish with chopped fresh parsley before serving, if desired.

14. Serve the Broccoli and Cheddar Stuffed Chicken hot, with any additional sauce spooned over the top

71. Tofu Pad Thai

Ingredients:
- 8 oz (225g) rice noodles
- 1 block (14 oz/400g) extra-firm tofu, drained and pressed
- 2 tablespoons vegetable oil
- 3 cloves garlic, minced
- 2 shallots, thinly sliced
- 2 cups bean sprouts
- 2 large eggs, beaten
- 1/4 cup roasted peanuts, chopped (optional, for garnish)
- 2 green onions, thinly sliced (for garnish)
- 1 lime, cut into wedges (for serving)
- Fresh cilantro (for garnish, optional)

For the sauce:
- 3 tablespoons tamarind paste
- 3 tablespoons soy sauce
- 2 tablespoons brown sugar
- 1 tablespoon rice vinegar
- 1 tablespoon lime juice
- 1 teaspoon sriracha sauce (adjust to taste)
- 2 tablespoons water

Instructions:

1. Cook the rice noodles according to the package instructions. Once cooked, rinse them under cold water, drain, and set aside.

2. Cut the pressed tofu into cubes.

3. In a small bowl, whisk together all the sauce ingredients: tamarind paste, soy sauce, brown sugar, rice vinegar, lime juice, sriracha sauce, and water. Set aside.

4. Heat vegetable oil in a large skillet or wok over medium-high heat.

5. Add minced garlic and thinly sliced shallots to the skillet. Stir-fry for about 1 minute until fragrant.

6. Add cubed tofu to the skillet and cook for about 5-7 minutes, stirring occasionally, until golden brown and crispy on all sides.

7. Push the tofu to one side of the skillet and pour beaten eggs into the other side. Scramble the eggs until cooked, then mix them with the tofu.

8. Add cooked rice noodles and bean sprouts to the skillet. Pour the prepared sauce over the noodles and tofu. Toss everything together until well combined.

9. Continue to stir-fry for another 2-3 minutes until heated through. Taste and adjust seasoning if needed.

10. Transfer the Tofu Pad Thai to serving plates or bowls. Garnish with chopped roasted peanuts, sliced green onions, fresh cilantro, and lime wedges. Serve the Tofu Pad Thai hot, with extra lime wedges on the side.

72. Creamy Sun-Dried Tomato Chicken

Ingredients:
- 4 boneless, skinless chicken breasts
- Salt and pepper to taste
- 2 tablespoons olive oil
- 4 cloves garlic, minced
- 1/2 cup sun-dried tomatoes, chopped
- 1 cup chicken broth
- 1 cup heavy cream
- 1 teaspoon dried basil
- 1/2 teaspoon dried oregano
- 1/4 teaspoon red pepper flakes (optional)
- 1/2 cup grated Parmesan cheese
- Fresh basil leaves, chopped (for garnish, optional)

Instructions:
1. Season the chicken breasts with salt and pepper to taste.

2. In a large skillet, heat olive oil over medium-high heat.

3. Add the seasoned chicken breasts to the skillet. Cook for about 5-6 minutes on each side, or until browned and cooked through. Remove the chicken from the skillet and set aside.

4. In the same skillet, add minced garlic and chopped sun-dried tomatoes. Cook for about 1-2 minutes until fragrant.

5. Pour chicken broth into the skillet and bring it to a simmer.

6. Stir in heavy cream, dried basil, dried oregano, and red pepper flakes (if using). Let the mixture simmer for about 2-3 minutes to allow the flavors to meld together.

7. Reduce the heat to low and stir in grated Parmesan cheese until melted and the sauce is creamy.

8. Return the cooked chicken breasts to the skillet and spoon the creamy sun-dried tomato sauce over them.

9. Let the chicken simmer in the sauce for another 2-3 minutes to heat through. Taste and adjust seasoning if needed.

10. Garnish with chopped fresh basil leaves before serving, if desired. Serve the Creamy Sun-Dried Tomato Chicken hot, over cooked pasta or rice.

73. Eggplant Parmesan

Ingredients:

- 1 large eggplant, sliced into 1/4-inch rounds
- Salt
- 1 cup all-purpose flour
- 2 eggs, beaten
- 1 cup breadcrumbs
- 1/2 cup grated Parmesan cheese
- 2 cups marinara sauce
- 1 cup shredded mozzarella cheese
- Fresh basil leaves, for garnish (optional)

Instructions:

1. Preheat the oven to 375°F (190°C).

2. Place the eggplant slices on a paper towel-lined baking sheet and sprinkle them with salt. Let them sit for about 15-20 minutes to release excess moisture. Pat them dry with paper towels.

3. Set up a dredging station with three shallow bowls: one with flour, one with beaten eggs, and one with a mixture of breadcrumbs and grated Parmesan cheese.

4. Dredge each eggplant slice in flour, then dip it in beaten eggs, and finally coat it in the breadcrumb mixture, pressing gently to adhere.

5. Heat a few tablespoons of olive oil in a large skillet over medium-high heat. Add the breaded eggplant slices to the skillet in a single layer, working in batches if necessary. Cook for about 2-3 minutes on each side until golden brown and crispy. Remove the cooked eggplant slices from the skillet and set aside.

6. Wipe out any excess oil from the skillet and spread a thin layer of marinara sauce on the bottom.

7. Arrange a layer of cooked eggplant slices on top of the marinara sauce.

8. Spoon more marinara sauce over the eggplant slices, then sprinkle shredded mozzarella cheese on top.

9. Repeat the layers until all the eggplant slices are used, ending with a layer of marinara sauce and shredded mozzarella cheese on top.

10. Place the skillet in the preheated oven and bake for about 20-25 minutes, or until the cheese is melted and bubbly.

11. Once cooked, remove the skillet from the oven and let it cool slightly. Garnish with fresh basil leaves before serving, if desired. Serve the Eggplant Parmesan hot as a delicious and comforting meal.

74. Skillet Corn and Zucchini

Ingredients:
- 2 tablespoons butter
- 2 medium zucchinis, diced
- 2 cups corn kernels (fresh, frozen, or canned)
- 1/4 teaspoon garlic powder
- Salt and pepper to taste
- 2 tablespoons chopped fresh parsley (optional, for garnish)

Instructions:
1. Heat butter in a large skillet over medium-high heat until melted.

2. Add diced zucchinis to the skillet and cook for about 5-7 minutes, stirring occasionally, until they start to soften.

3. Stir in corn kernels and continue to cook for another 5-7 minutes, or until the corn is heated through and tender.

4. Sprinkle garlic powder over the skillet and season with salt and pepper to taste. Stir well to combine.

5. Cook for another 1-2 minutes until the flavors meld together.

6. Taste and adjust seasoning if needed.

7. Garnish with chopped fresh parsley before serving, if desired.

8. Serve the Skillet Corn and Zucchini hot as a delicious side dish.

Enjoy your delicious and easy single-skillet Skillet Corn and Zucchini!

75. Miso Glazed Salmon

Ingredients:
- 4 salmon fillets (about 6 oz each)
- Salt and pepper to taste
- 2 tablespoons miso paste
- 2 tablespoons soy sauce
- 2 tablespoons honey
- 2 cloves garlic, minced
- 1 tablespoon grated ginger
- 1 tablespoon sesame oil
- 1 tablespoon vegetable oil
- ptional garnish: sliced green onions, sesame seeds

Instructions:

1. Season the salmon fillets with salt and pepper to taste on both sides.

2. In a small bowl, whisk together miso paste, soy sauce, honey, minced garlic, grated ginger, and sesame oil to make the glaze.

3. Heat vegetable oil in a large skillet over medium-high heat.

4. Place the salmon fillets in the skillet, skin-side down. Cook for about 3-4 minutes until the skin is crispy.

5. Flip the salmon fillets and pour the miso glaze over them.

6. Continue to cook for another 3-4 minutes, spooning the glaze over the salmon occasionaly, until the salmon is cooked through and glazed.

7. Remove the skillet from the heat.

8. Garnish the Miso Glazed Salmon with sliced green onions and sesame seeds, if desired.

9. Serve the salmon hot, accompanied by your favorite side dishes, such as steamed rice and vegetables.

Enjoy your delicious and easy single-skillet Miso Glazed Salmon!

76. Chickpea and Spinach Curry

Ingredients:

- 2 tablespoons olive oil
- 1 onion, finely chopped
- 3 cloves garlic, minced
- 1 tablespoon grated ginger
- 1 tablespoon curry powder
- 1 teaspoon ground cumin
- 1 teaspoon ground coriander
- 1/2 teaspoon turmeric
- 1/4 teaspoon cayenne pepper (adjust to taste)
- 1 (14 oz) can diced tomatoes
- 2 (14 oz) cans chickpeas, drained and rinsed
- 1 (14 oz) can coconut milk
- Salt and pepper to taste
- 4 cups fresh spinach leaves
- Fresh cilantro leaves, for garnish
- Cooked rice or naan bread, for serving

Instructions:

1. Heat olive oil in a large skillet over medium heat.

2. Add finely chopped onion to the skillet and cook for about 5 minutes until softened.

3. Stir in minced garlic and grated ginger. Cook for another 1-2 minutes until fragrant.

4. Add curry powder, ground cumin, ground coriander, turmeric, and cayenne pepper to the skillet. Stir well to coat the onion mixture with the spices. Cook for about 1 minute until aromatic.

5. Pour diced tomatoes (with their juices) into the skillet. Stir to combine with the onion and spice mixture.

6. Add drained and rinsed chickpeas to the skillet. Stir well to coat the chickpeas with the tomato mixture.

7. Pour coconut milk into the skillet and stir to combine. Bring the mixture to a simmer.

8. Let the curry simmer for about 10-15 minutes, stirring occasionally, until the flavors meld together and the sauce thickens slightly.

9. Season the curry with salt and pepper to taste.

10. Stir in fresh spinach leaves and let them wilt into the curry for about 2-3 minutes.

11. Taste and adjust seasoning if needed.

12. Garnish the Chickpea and Spinach Curry with fresh cilantro leaves before serving. Serve the curry hot with cooked rice or naan bread.

77. Chicken and Mushroom Skillet

Ingredients:
- 4 boneless, skinless chicken breasts
- Salt and pepper to taste
- 2 tablespoons olive oil
- 8 ounces (225g) mushrooms, sliced
- 3 cloves garlic, minced
- 1 teaspoon dried thyme
- 1 teaspoon dried rosemary
- 1/2 cup chicken broth
- 1/2 cup heavy cream
- 2 tablespoons chopped fresh parsley (optional, for garnish)

Instructions:

1. Season the chicken breasts with salt and pepper to taste on both sides.

2. In a large skillet, heat olive oil over medium-high heat.

3. Add the seasoned chicken breasts to the skillet. Cook for about 5-6 minutes on each side, or until browned and cooked through. Remove the chicken from the skillet and set aside.

4. In the same skillet, add sliced mushrooms. Cook for about 5-7 minutes, stirring occasionally, until the mushrooms are golden brown and tender.

5. Add minced garlic, dried thyme, and dried rosemary to the skillet. Cook for another 1-2 minutes until fragrant.

6. Pour chicken broth into the skillet and stir to deglaze the bottom of the pan, scraping up any browned bits.

7. Stir in heavy cream and bring the mixture to a simmer.

8. Return the cooked chicken breasts to the skillet, nestling them into the mushroom sauce.

9. Let the chicken simmer in the sauce for another 2-3 minutes to heat through.

10. Taste and adjust seasoning if needed.

11. Garnish with chopped fresh parsley before serving, if desired.

12. Serve the Chicken and Mushroom Skillet hot, accompanied by your favorite side dishes.

78. Lemon Herb Quinoa

Ingredients:
- 1 cup quinoa, rinsed and drained
- 2 cups vegetable broth or water
- 2 tablespoons olive oil
- 2 cloves garlic, minced
- Zest of 1 lemon
- Juice of 1 lemon
- 1 teaspoon dried thyme
- 1 teaspoon dried rosemary
- Salt and pepper to taste
- 2 tablespoons chopped fresh parsley (optional, for garnish)

Instructions:

1. In a large skillet, heat olive oil over medium heat.

2. Add minced garlic to the skillet and cook for about 1 minute until fragrant.

3. Add rinsed and drained quinoa to the skillet. Stir to toast the quinoa for about 2-3 minutes.

4. Pour vegetable broth or water into the skillet. Stir in lemon zest, lemon juice, dried thyme, and dried rosemary.

5. Season with salt and pepper to taste. Stir well to combine.

6. Bring the mixture to a boil, then reduce the heat to low. Cover and let the quinoa simmer for about 15-20 minutes, or until the liquid is absorbed and the quinoa is tender.

7. Once the quinoa is cooked, fluff it with a fork.

8. Taste and adjust seasoning if needed.

9. Garnish with chopped fresh parsley before serving, if desired.

10. Serve the Lemon Herb Quinoa hot as a delicious and nutritious side dish.

Enjoy your delicious and easy single-skillet Lemon Herb Quinoa!

79. One-Pot Sausage and Tortellini

Ingredients:
- 1 lb (450g) Italian sausage, casings removed
- 1 tablespoon olive oil
- 1 onion, diced
- 3 cloves garlic, minced
- 1 (14 oz) can diced tomatoes
- 4 cups chicken broth
- 1 teaspoon dried basil
- 1 teaspoon dried oregano
- 1/2 teaspoon red pepper flakes (optional)
- Salt and pepper to taste
- 1 (9 oz) package refrigerated cheese tortellini
- 2 cups baby spinach leaves
- 1/2 cup grated Parmesan cheese
- Chopped fresh parsley for garnish (optional)

Instructions:

1. Heat olive oil in a large skillet over medium heat. Add Italian sausage, breaking it up with a spoon, and cook until browned and cooked through, about 5-7 minutes.

2. Add diced onion to the skillet and cook for about 3-4 minutes until softened.

3. Stir in minced garlic and cook for another 1-2 minutes until fragrant.

4. Add diced tomatoes (with their juices), chicken broth, dried basil, dried oregano, red pepper flakes (if using), salt, and pepper to the skillet. Stir to combine.

5. Bring the mixture to a boil, then reduce the heat to low and let it simmer for about 10 minutes to allow the flavors to meld together.

6. Stir in refrigerated cheese tortellini and baby spinach leaves. Cook for about 5-7 minutes, or until the tortellini is cooked through and the spinach is wilted.

7. Once the tortellini is cooked, remove the skillet from the heat.

8. Stir in grated Parmesan cheese until melted and the sauce is creamy.

9. Taste and adjust seasoning if needed.

10. Garnish with chopped fresh parsley before serving, if desired. Serve the One-Pot Sausage and Tortellini hot, with extra Parmesan cheese on top

80. Spicy Tofu Stir-Fry

Ingredients:

- 1 block (14 oz/400g) firm tofu, pressed and cubed
- 2 tablespoons soy sauce
- 1 tablespoon sriracha sauce (adjust to taste)
- 1 tablespoon rice vinegar
- 1 tablespoon honey or maple syrup
- 1 tablespoon sesame oil
- 2 tablespoons vegetable oil
- 3 cloves garlic, minced
- 1 tablespoon minced ginger
- 1 bell pepper, thinly sliced
- 1 small onion, thinly sliced
- 1 cup broccoli florets
- 1 carrot, thinly sliced
- Cooked rice, for serving
- Sesame seeds and chopped green onions, for garnish (optional)

Instructions:

1. In a small bowl, whisk together soy sauce, sriracha sauce, rice vinegar, honey or maple syrup, and sesame oil. Set aside.

2. Heat vegetable oil in a large skillet or wok over medium-high heat.

3. Add minced garlic and minced ginger to the skillet. Stir-fry for about 1 minute until fragrant.

4. Add cubed tofu to the skillet. Cook for about 5-7 minutes, stirring occasionally, until the tofu is golden brown and crispy on all sides.

5. Add thinly sliced bell pepper, onion, broccoli florets, and thinly sliced carrot to the skillet. Stir-fry for about 3-4 minutes, or until the vegetables are tender-crisp.

6. Pour the prepared sauce over the tofu and vegetables in the skillet. Stir well to coat everything evenly.

7. Cook for another 2-3 minutes, stirring occasionally, until the sauce thickens slightly and coats the tofu and vegetables.

8. Taste and adjust seasoning if needed.

9. Once cooked, remove the skillet from the heat.

10. Serve the Spicy Tofu Stir-Fry hot over cooked rice.

11. Garnish with sesame seeds and chopped green onions, if desired.

Enjoy your delicious and easy single-skillet Spicy Tofu Stir-Fry!

81. Creamy Cajun Chicken Pasta

Ingredients:

- 8 oz (225g) penne pasta
- 2 boneless, skinless chicken breasts, thinly sliced
- 2 tablespoons Cajun seasoning
- 2 tablespoons olive oil
- 2 cloves garlic, minced
- 1 bell pepper, thinly sliced
- 1 small onion, thinly sliced
- 1 cup sliced mushrooms
- 1 cup chicken broth
- 1 cup heavy cream
- 1/2 cup grated Parmesan cheese
- Salt and pepper to taste
- Fresh parsley, chopped (for garnish)
- Lemon wedges (for serving, optional)

Instructions:

1. Cook the penne pasta according to the package instructions until al dente. Drain and set aside.

2. Season the thinly sliced chicken breasts with Cajun seasoning.

3. In a large skillet, heat olive oil over medium-high heat. Add the seasoned chicken breasts to the skillet and cook for about 5-7 minutes on each side until cooked through and browned. Remove the chicken from the skillet and set aside.

4. In the same skillet, add minced garlic, thinly sliced bell pepper, onion, and sliced mushrooms. Cook for about 5 minutes until the vegetables are softened.

5. Pour chicken broth into the skillet and deglaze the bottom, scraping up any browned bits.

6. Stir in heavy cream and bring the mixture to a simmer. Add cooked penne pasta to the skillet and stir to combine with the sauce.

7. Stir in grated Parmesan cheese until melted and the sauce is creamy. Season with salt and pepper to taste.

8. Return the cooked chicken breasts to the skillet and let them heat through for another 2-3 minutes.

9. Once everything is heated through and the sauce has thickened, remove the skillet from the heat.

10. Garnish with chopped fresh parsley. Serve the Creamy Cajun Chicken Pasta hot, with lemon wedges on the side for squeezing over the pasta, if desired.

Enjoy your delicious and easy single-skillet Creamy Cajun Chicken Pasta!

82. Vegetarian Chili Mac

Ingredients:

- 8 oz (225g) elbow macaroni pasta
- 1 tablespoon olive oil
- 1 onion, diced
- 2 cloves garlic, minced
- 1 bell pepper, diced
- 1 (15 oz) can black beans, drained and rinsed
- 1 (15 oz) can kidney beans, drained and rinsed
- 1 (15 oz) can diced tomatoes
- 1 tablespoon chili powder
- 1 teaspoon cumin
- 2 cups vegetable broth
- 1/2 teaspoon paprika
- Salt and pepper to taste
- 1 cup shredded cheddar cheese (optional, for topping)
- Chopped fresh cilantro or green onions, for garnish (optional)

Instructions:

1. In a large skillet, heat olive oil over medium heat. Add diced onion and cook for about 3-4 minutes until softened.

2. Add minced garlic and diced bell pepper to the skillet. Cook for another 2-3 minutes until the vegetables are tender.

3. Stir in chili powder, cumin, paprika, salt, and pepper. Cook for about 1 minute until fragrant.

4. Pour diced tomatoes (with their juices) and vegetable broth into the skillet. Stir to combine.

5. Add elbow macaroni pasta to the skillet and stir well to combine with the vegetable mixture.

6. Bring the mixture to a simmer, then reduce the heat to low. Cover and let it simmer for about 12-15 minutes, stirring occasionally, until the pasta is cooked and the sauce is thickened.

7. Stir in drained and rinsed black beans and kidney beans. Cook for another 2-3 minutes until heated through.

8. Taste and adjust seasoning if needed.

9. Once everything is cooked through and the sauce has thickened, remove the skillet from the heat.

10. If desired, sprinkle shredded cheddar cheese over the top of the Vegetarian Chili Mac and let it melt from the residual heat of the skillet.

11. Garnish with chopped fresh cilantro or green onions before serving, if desired. Serve the Vegetarian Chili Mac hot, with additional toppings like sour cream or avocado if desired.

83. Skillet Garlic Butter Shrimp

Ingredients:
- 1 lb (450g) large shrimp, peeled and deveined
- Salt and pepper to taste
- 2 tablespoons olive oil
- 4 tablespoons unsalted butter
- 4 cloves garlic, minced
- 1/2 teaspoon red pepper flakes (optional)
- 2 tablespoons chopped fresh parsley
- 1 tablespoon lemon juice

Instructions:

1. Pat the shrimp dry with paper towels and season with salt and pepper to taste.

2. Heat olive oil in a large skillet over medium-high heat.

3. Add the shrimp to the skillet in a single layer. Cook for about 1-2 minutes on each side until pink and opaque. Remove the shrimp from the skillet and set aside.

4. In the same skillet, add unsalted butter. Once melted, add minced garlic and red pepper flakes (if using). Cook for about 1 minute until fragrant.

5. Return the cooked shrimp to the skillet. Stir well to coat the shrimp with the garlic butter sauce.

6. Cook for another 1-2 minutes until the shrimp are heated through.

7. Stir in chopped fresh parsley and lemon juice. Cook for another 1 minute, stirring continuously.

8. Taste and adjust seasoning if needed.

9. Once everything is heated through and coated in the garlic butter sauce, remove the skillet from the heat.

10. Serve the Skillet Garlic Butter Shrimp hot, with cooked rice, pasta, or crusty bread on the side.

Enjoy your delicious and easy single-skillet Skillet Garlic Butter Shrimp!

84. Greek Lemon Chicken and Potatoes

Ingredients:

- 4 bone-in, skin-on chicken thighs
- Salt and pepper to taste
- 1 tablespoon dried oregano
- 1 tablespoon dried thyme
- 4 tablespoons olive oil, divided
- 4 medium potatoes, peeled and cut into wedges
- 4 cloves garlic, minced
- 1/2 cup chicken broth
- Juice of 2 lemons
- Zest of 1 lemon
- 1/2 cup pitted Kalamata olives
- 1/4 cup chopped fresh parsley (for garnish)
- Lemon slices (for garnish)

Instructions:

1. Preheat the oven to 400°F (200°C).

2. Season the chicken thighs with salt, pepper, dried oregano, and dried thyme.

3. In a large oven-safe skillet, heat 2 tablespoons of olive oil over medium-high heat. Add the chicken thighs to the skillet, skin-side down. Cook for about 5-7 minutes until the skin is golden brown and crispy. Flip the chicken thighs and cook for another 2-3 minutes on the other side. Remove the chicken from the skillet and set aside.

4. In the same skillet, add the remaining 2 tablespoons of olive oil. Add the potato wedges to the skillet and cook for about 5-7 minutes until they start to brown.

5. Add minced garlic to the skillet and cook for another 1 minute until fragrant.

6. Pour chicken broth, lemon juice, and lemon zest into the skillet. Stir to combine.

7. Return the cooked chicken thighs to the skillet, nestling them among the potatoes.

8. Scatter Kalamata olives over the chicken and potatoes.

9. Transfer the skillet to the preheated oven and bake for about 25-30 minutes, or until the chicken is cooked through and the potatoes are tender.

10. Once cooked, remove the skillet from the oven.

11. Garnish the Greek Lemon Chicken and Potatoes with chopped fresh parsley and lemon slices before serving.

12. Serve hot and enjoy your delicious and easy single-skillet Greek Lemon Chicken and Potatoes!

85. Tomato Basil Pasta

Ingredients:

- 8 oz (225g) pasta (such as spaghetti or penne)
- 2 tablespoons olive oil
- 4 cloves garlic, minced
- 1 (14 oz/400g) can diced tomatoes
- 1 teaspoon dried basil (or 1 tablespoon chopped fresh basil)
- Salt and pepper to taste
- 1/4 teaspoon red pepper flakes (optional)
- Grated Parmesan cheese, for serving
- Chopped fresh basil, for garnish

Instructions:

1. Cook the pasta according to the package instructions until al dente. Reserve about 1/2 cup of pasta water, then drain the pasta and set it aside.

2. In the same skillet, heat olive oil over medium heat.

3. Add minced garlic to the skillet and cook for about 1 minute until fragrant.

4. Pour diced tomatoes (with their juices) into the skillet. Stir well to combine with the garlic.

5. Add dried basil (or chopped fresh basil), salt, pepper, and red pepper flakes (if using). Stir to combine.

6. Let the tomato mixture simmer for about 5-7 minutes, stirring occasionally, until it thickens slightly.

7. If the sauce becomes too thick, you can add a splash of reserved pasta water to thin it out.

8. Once the sauce has reached your desired consistency, add the cooked pasta to the skillet. Toss well to coat the pasta evenly with the sauce.

9. Taste and adjust seasoning if needed.

10. Serve the Tomato Basil Pasta hot, garnished with grated Parmesan cheese and chopped fresh basil.

Enjoy your delicious and easy single-skillet Tomato Basil Pasta!

86. Szechuan Tofu and Vegetable Stir-Fry

Ingredients:

- 14 oz (400g) firm tofu, drained and cubed
- 2 tablespoons soy sauce
- 2 tablespoons cornstarch
- 2 tablespoons vegetable oil
- 2 cloves garlic, minced
- 1 tablespoon minced ginger
- 1 bell pepper, thinly sliced
- 1 carrot, thinly sliced
- 1 cup broccoli florets
- 1 cup snap peas
- 1/4 cup sliced green onions (scallions), for garnish

For the Sauce:

- 1/4 cup soy sauce
- 2 tablespoons hoisin sauce
- 1 tablespoon rice vinegar
- 1 tablespoon brown sugar
- 1 teaspoon Szechuan peppercorns (optional, for extra heat)
- 1 teaspoon chili garlic sauce (adjust to taste)

Instructions:

1. In a bowl, mix together 2 tablespoons of soy sauce and cornstarch. Add the cubed tofu and toss to coat. Set aside to marinate for about 10 minutes.

2. In a separate bowl, whisk together all the ingredients for the sauce - soy sauce, hoisin sauce, rice vinegar, brown sugar, Szechuan peppercorns (if using), and chili garlic sauce. Set aside.

3. Heat vegetable oil in a large skillet or wok over medium-high heat. Add the marinated tofu cubes and cook until golden brown and crispy on all sides, about 5-7 minutes. Remove tofu from the skillet and set aside.

4. In the same skillet, add minced garlic and minced ginger. Stir-fry for about 1 minute until fragrant.

5. Add sliced bell pepper, carrot, broccoli florets, and snap peas to the skillet. Stir-fry for about 5-7 minutes until the vegetables are tender-crisp.

6. Return the cooked tofu to the skillet and pour the sauce over the tofu and vegetables. Stir well to combine.

7. Cook for another 2-3 minutes, allowing the sauce to thicken and coat the tofu and vegetables.

8. Taste and adjust seasoning if needed. Once everything is heated through and coated in the sauce, remove the skillet from the heat.

10. Serve the Szechuan Tofu and Vegetable Stir-Fry hot, garnished with sliced green onions.

87. Cheeseburger Skillet

Ingredients:
- 1 lb (450g) ground beef
- 1 onion, diced
- 2 cloves garlic, minced
- 1 teaspoon Worcestershire sauce
- Salt and pepper to taste
- 1 cup beef broth
- 1 (14 oz) can diced tomatoes
- 2 cups elbow macaroni
- 1 cup shredded cheddar cheese
- 1/4 cup chopped dill pickles
- Optional toppings: chopped tomatoes, shredded lettuce, diced onions, ketchup, mustard

Instructions:

1. In a large skillet, cook ground beef over medium-high heat until browned, breaking it up with a spoon as it cooks.

2. Add diced onion and minced garlic to the skillet with the browned beef. Cook for about 3-4 minutes until the onions are softened.

3. Stir in Worcestershire sauce, salt, and pepper to taste.

4. Pour beef broth and diced tomatoes (with their juices) into the skillet. Stir well to combine.

5. Add elbow macaroni to the skillet and stir to combine with the beef mixture.

6. Bring the mixture to a simmer, then cover the skillet and reduce the heat to medium-low. Let it simmer for about 10-12 minutes, stirring occasionally, until the macaroni is cooked and the sauce has thickened.

7. Once the macaroni is cooked, sprinkle shredded cheddar cheese over the top of the skillet. Cover and let it sit for about 1-2 minutes until the cheese is melted.

8. Remove the skillet from the heat and sprinkle chopped dill pickles over the top of the cheeseburger skillet.

9. Serve the Cheeseburger Skillet hot, with optional toppings like chopped tomatoes, shredded lettuce, diced onions, ketchup, and mustard.

88. Lemon Garlic Butter Scallops

Ingredients:

- 1 lb (450g) large sea scallops, patted dry
- Salt and pepper to taste
- 2 tablespoons unsalted butter
- 2 tablespoons olive oil
- 4 cloves garlic, minced
- Zest of 1 lemon
- Juice of 1 lemon
- 2 tablespoons chopped fresh parsley
- Lemon wedges, for serving
- Chopped fresh parsley, for garnish (optional)

Instructions:

1. Pat the scallops dry with paper towels and season them with salt and pepper on both sides.

2. In a large skillet, heat 1 tablespoon of butter and 1 tablespoon of olive oil over medium-high heat.

3. Once the skillet is hot, add the scallops to the skillet in a single layer, making sure they are not overcrowded. Cook the scallops for about 2-3 minutes on each side until they are golden brown and caramelized on the outside, and opaque in the center. Be careful not to overcook them, as scallops can become tough if cooked for too long. Cook in batches if necessary.

4. Remove the cooked scallops from the skillet and set them aside on a plate. Cover them with foil to keep warm.

5. In the same skillet, add the remaining butter and olive oil. Add minced garlic to the skillet and cook for about 1 minute until fragrant.

6. Add lemon zest and lemon juice to the skillet. Stir well to combine with the garlic and butter mixture.

7. Return the cooked scallops to the skillet and toss them gently in the lemon garlic butter sauce to coat.

8. Sprinkle chopped fresh parsley over the scallops and stir gently to combine. Once the scallops are heated through and coated in the sauce, remove the skillet from the heat.

9. Serve the Lemon Garlic Butter Scallops hot, garnished with additional chopped fresh parsley and lemon wedges on the side.

89. Crispy Tofu with Peanut Sauce

Ingredients:

For the Crispy Tofu:
- 14 oz (400g) firm tofu, pressed and cut into cubes
- 2 tablespoons cornstarch
- 2 tablespoons soy sauce
- 2 tablespoons sesame oil
- Salt and pepper to taste
- 2 tablespoons vegetable oil, for frying

For Garnish:
- Chopped green onions
- Sesame seeds
- Crushed peanuts
- Sliced red chili (optional)

For the Peanut Sauce:
- 1/4 cup creamy peanut butter
- 2 tablespoons soy sauce
- 1 tablespoon rice vinegar
- 1 tablespoon maple syrup or honey
- 1 teaspoon sesame oil
- 1 clove garlic, minced
- 1/4 teaspoon red pepper flakes (optional)
- 2-4 tablespoons water, to thin the sauce

Instructions:

1. In a small bowl, mix together cornstarch, soy sauce, sesame oil, salt, and pepper to create a marinade for the tofu.

2. Toss the tofu cubes in the marinade until evenly coated. Allow the tofu to marinate for at least 15-20 minutes.

3. In the meantime, prepare the peanut sauce. In a small saucepan over low heat, combine peanut butter, soy sauce, rice vinegar, maple syrup or honey, sesame oil, minced garlic, and red pepper flakes. Stir well until smooth and creamy. If the sauce is too thick, add water, 1 tablespoon at a time, until desired consistency is reached. Keep warm over low heat.

4. Heat vegetable oil in a large skillet over medium-high heat. Once hot, add the marinated tofu cubes in a single layer, ensuring they are not overcrowded. Cook for about 3-4 minutes on each side, or until golden and crispy. You may need to work in batches.

5. Once crispy and golden brown, remove the tofu from the skillet and place it on a paper towel-lined plate to drain any excess oil.

6. Serve the crispy tofu drizzled with the prepared peanut sauce. Garnish with chopped green onions, sesame seeds, crushed peanuts, and sliced red chili, if desired.

7. Enjoy your delicious and easy single-skillet Crispy Tofu with Peanut Sauce!

90. Skillet Sausage and Peppers Pasta

Ingredients:

- 8 oz (225g) pasta (such as penne or fusilli)
- 1 tablespoon olive oil
- 4 Italian sausages, casings removed
- 1 onion, thinly sliced
- 2 bell peppers (red, green, or yellow), thinly sliced
- 3 cloves garlic, minced
- 1 (14 oz/400g) can diced tomatoes
- 1 teaspoon dried oregano
- 1 teaspoon dried basil
- Salt and pepper to taste
- 1/4 cup grated Parmesan cheese, plus extra for serving
- Fresh basil leaves, torn, for garnish

Instructions:

1. Cook the pasta according to the package instructions until al dente. Drain and set aside.

2. In a large skillet, heat olive oil over medium heat.

3. Add the Italian sausages to the skillet, breaking them up with a spoon as they cook. Cook until browned and cooked through, about 5-7 minutes.

4. Add the thinly sliced onion and bell peppers to the skillet. Cook, stirring occasionally, until the vegetables are softened, about 5 minutes.

5. Add the minced garlic to the skillet and cook for an additional minute until fragrant.

6. Stir in the diced tomatoes (with their juices), dried oregano, and dried basil. Season with salt and pepper to taste.

7. Allow the mixture to simmer for about 5-7 minutes to allow the flavors to meld together.

8. Add the cooked pasta to the skillet and toss to combine with the sausage and peppers mixture.

9. Stir in the grated Parmesan cheese until melted and the sauce is creamy. Taste and adjust seasoning if necessary.

10. Once everything is heated through and well combined, remove the skillet from the heat.

11. Serve the Skillet Sausage and Peppers Pasta hot, garnished with extra grated Parmesan cheese and torn fresh basil leaves.

12. Enjoy your delicious and easy single-skillet Skillet Sausage and Peppers Pasta!

91. Spinach and Ricotta Stuffed Chicken

Ingredients:

- 4 boneless, skinless chicken breasts
- Salt and pepper to taste
- 1 cup fresh spinach, chopped
- 1/2 cup ricotta cheese
- 1/4 cup grated Parmesan cheese
- 2 cloves garlic, minced
- 1 tablespoon olive oil
- 1 cup marinara sauce
- 1/2 cup shredded mozzarella cheese
- Fresh basil leaves, for garnish (optional)

Instructions:

1. Preheat your oven to 375°F (190°C).

2. Use a sharp knife to carefully slice a pocket into the side of each chicken breast, being careful not to cut all the way through.

3. Season the inside of each chicken breast with salt and pepper.

4. In a mixing bowl, combine chopped spinach, ricotta cheese, grated Parmesan cheese, and minced garlic. Mix until well combined.

5. Stuff each chicken breast with the spinach and ricotta mixture, dividing it evenly among them.

6. In a large oven-safe skillet, heat olive oil over medium-high heat.

7. Once the skillet is hot, add the stuffed chicken breasts to the skillet. Cook for about 5-6 minutes on each side, or until they are golden brown and cooked through.

8. Remove the skillet from the heat and spoon marinara sauce over each chicken breast.

9. Sprinkle shredded mozzarella cheese over the top of each chicken breast.

10. Transfer the skillet to the preheated oven and bake for about 10-12 minutes, or until the cheese is melted and bubbly.

11. Once cooked through, remove the skillet from the oven.

12. Garnish the Spinach and Ricotta Stuffed Chicken with fresh basil leaves, if desired.

13. Serve hot, with any remaining marinara sauce from the skillet spooned over the top.

Enjoy your delicious and easy single-skillet Spinach and Ricotta Stuffed Chicken!

92. Vegetable Pad Thai

Ingredients:

- 8 oz (225g) rice noodles
- 2 tablespoons vegetable oil
- 2 cloves garlic, minced
- 1 small onion, thinly sliced
- 1 bell pepper, thinly sliced
- 1 carrot, julienned or thinly sliced
- 2 cups bean sprouts
- 2 green onions, chopped
- 1/4 cup chopped peanuts, for garnish
- Lime wedges, for serving
- Fresh cilantro leaves, for garnish

For the Sauce:

- 1/4 cup soy sauce
- 2 tablespoons tamarind paste (or substitute with rice vinegar)
- 2 tablespoons brown sugar (adjust to taste)
- 1 tablespoon fish sauce (optional, for non-vegetarian version)
- 1 tablespoon lime juice

Instructions:

1. Cook the rice noodles according to the package instructions until they are al dente. Drain and set aside.

2. In a small bowl, mix together all the ingredients for the sauce: soy sauce, tamarind paste (or rice vinegar), brown sugar, fish sauce (if using), and lime juice. Set aside.

3. Heat vegetable oil in a large skillet or wok over medium-high heat.

4. Add minced garlic to the skillet and cook for about 30 seconds until fragrant.

5. Add thinly sliced onion, bell pepper, and julienned carrot to the skillet. Stir-fry for about 3-4 minutes until the vegetables are tender-crisp.

6. Add the cooked rice noodles and bean sprouts to the skillet. Pour the sauce over the noodles and vegetables. Toss well to combine and coat everything evenly in the sauce.

7. Continue to stir-fry for another 2-3 minutes until everything is heated through and well combined.

8. Taste and adjust seasoning if necessary, adding more soy sauce, brown sugar, or lime juice as desired.

9. Once everything is cooked through, remove the skillet from the heat.

10. Serve the Vegetable Pad Thai hot, garnished with chopped green onions, chopped peanuts, lime wedges, and fresh cilantro leaves.

11. Enjoy your delicious and easy single-skillet Vegetable Pad Thai!

93. Creamy Pesto Gnocchi

Ingredients:
- 17.6 oz (500g) package of store-bought gnocchi
- 2 tablespoons olive oil
- 2 cloves garlic, minced
- 1/2 cup sun-dried tomatoes, chopped
- 1/4 cup store-bought pesto sauce
- 1/2 cup heavy cream
- Salt and pepper to taste
- Grated Parmesan cheese, for garnish
- Fresh basil leaves, chopped, for garnish (optional)

Instructions:

1. Cook the gnocchi according to the package instructions until they float to the surface. Drain and set aside.

2. In a large skillet, heat olive oil over medium heat.

3. Add minced garlic to the skillet and sauté for about 1 minute until fragrant.

4. Add chopped sun-dried tomatoes to the skillet and cook for an additional 1-2 minutes.

5. Stir in the cooked gnocchi and pesto sauce, tossing to coat the gnocchi evenly.

6. Pour in the heavy cream and stir well to combine. Allow the mixture to simmer gently for 2-3 minutes until the sauce thickens slightly.

7. Season with salt and pepper to taste.

8. Once the sauce has reached your desired consistency, remove the skillet from the heat.

9. Serve the Creamy Pesto Gnocchi hot, garnished with grated Parmesan cheese and chopped fresh basil leaves if desired.

10. Enjoy your delicious and easy single-skillet Creamy Pesto Gnocchi!

94. One-Pan Honey Mustard Chicken and Potatoes

Ingredients:
- 4 bone-in, skin-on chicken thighs
- Salt and pepper to taste
- 1 lb (450g) baby potatoes, halved
- 2 tablespoons olive oil
- 3 tablespoons whole grain mustard
- 2 tablespoons honey
- 2 cloves garlic, minced
- 1 teaspoon dried thyme (or 1 tablespoon chopped fresh thyme)
- 1 tablespoon chopped fresh parsley, for garnish (optional)

Instructions:
1. Preheat your oven to 400°F (200°C).

2. Season the chicken thighs with salt and pepper on both sides.

3. In a small bowl, whisk together olive oil, whole grain mustard, honey, minced garlic, and dried thyme.

4. In a large oven-safe skillet, heat a bit of olive oil over medium-high heat. Add the chicken thighs to the skillet, skin-side down, and cook for about 5 minutes until they're golden brown. Flip them and cook for another 3 minutes. Remove the chicken from the skillet and set it aside.

5. In the same skillet, add the halved baby potatoes. Cook for about 5 minutes until they start to brown.

6. Return the chicken thighs to the skillet, nestling them among the potatoes.

7. Pour the honey mustard sauce over the chicken and potatoes, ensuring everything is coated evenly.

8. Transfer the skillet to the preheated oven and bake for about 25-30 minutes until the chicken is cooked through and the potatoes are tender.

9. Once cooked, remove the skillet from the oven.

10. Serve the One-Pan Honey Mustard Chicken and Potatoes hot, garnished with chopped fresh parsley if desired.

11. Enjoy your delicious and easy single-skillet meal!

95. Mushroom and Spinach Skillet Pizza

Ingredients:

- 1 pre-made pizza dough (store-bought or homemade)
- 1 tablespoon olive oil
- 2 cloves garlic, minced
- 8 oz (225g) mushrooms, sliced
- 2 cups fresh spinach leaves
- 1 cup shredded mozzarella cheese
- 1/4 cup grated Parmesan cheese
- Salt and pepper to taste
- Red pepper flakes (optional, for added heat)
- Fresh basil leaves, chopped, for garnish (optional)

Instructions:

1. Preheat your oven to 425°F (220°C).

2. Roll out the pizza dough on a lightly floured surface to fit the size of your skillet.

3. Heat olive oil in an oven-safe skillet over medium heat.

4. Add minced garlic to the skillet and cook for about 1 minute until fragrant.

5. Add sliced mushrooms to the skillet and cook for about 5 minutes until they start to brown.

6. Add fresh spinach leaves to the skillet and cook for an additional 2-3 minutes until they are wilted. Season with salt and pepper to taste.

7. Push the mushroom and spinach mixture to the edges of the skillet, creating space in the center.

8. Place the rolled-out pizza dough in the center of the skillet, pressing it down gently to fit.

9. Spread shredded mozzarella cheese evenly over the pizza dough, followed by the cooked mushroom and spinach mixture.

10. Sprinkle grated Parmesan cheese over the top, along with red pepper flakes if desired.

11. Transfer the skillet to the preheated oven and bake for about 15-20 minutes until the crust is golden brown and the cheese is melted and bubbly.

12. Once cooked, remove the skillet from the oven.

13. Garnish the Mushroom and Spinach Skillet Pizza with chopped fresh basil leaves if desired.. Slice and serve hot.

96. Tofu and Vegetable Curry

Ingredients:

- 14 oz (400g) firm tofu, drained and cubed
- 2 tablespoons vegetable oil
- 1 onion, chopped
- 2 cloves garlic, minced
- 1 tablespoon grated ginger
- 2 tablespoons curry powder
- 1 teaspoon ground cumin
- 1 teaspoon ground coriander
- 1/2 teaspoon turmeric powder
- 1 can (14 oz/400g) coconut milk
- 1 cup vegetable broth
- 2 cups mixed vegetables (such as bell peppers, carrots, broccoli, cauliflower)
- Salt and pepper to taste
- Cooked rice or naan bread, for serving
- Fresh cilantro leaves, for garnish (optional)

Instructions:

1. Heat vegetable oil in a large skillet over medium heat.

2. Add chopped onion to the skillet and cook for about 3-4 minutes until softened.

3. Add minced garlic and grated ginger to the skillet. Cook for another 1-2 minutes until fragrant.

4. Stir in curry powder, ground cumin, ground coriander, and turmeric powder. Cook for about 1 minute until the spices are fragrant.

5. Add cubed tofu to the skillet and stir to coat with the spice mixture.

6. Pour in coconut milk and vegetable broth. Stir well to combine.

7. Bring the mixture to a simmer and let it cook for about 5 minutes, allowing the flavors to meld together.

8. Add mixed vegetables to the skillet. Stir well to combine.

9. Cover the skillet and let the curry simmer for another 10-15 minutes, or until the vegetables are tender and the tofu is heated through.

10. Taste and adjust seasoning with salt and pepper as needed.

11. Once everything is cooked through, remove the skillet from the heat.

12. Serve the Tofu and Vegetable Curry hot, with cooked rice or naan bread.

13. Garnish with fresh cilantro leaves if desired.

97. One-Pot Creamy Garlic Chicken Pasta

Ingredients:

- 8 oz (225g) linguine pasta
- 2 tablespoons olive oil
- 2 boneless, skinless chicken breasts, cut into bite-sized pieces
- Salt and pepper to taste
- 4 cloves garlic, minced
- 2 cups chicken broth
- 1 cup heavy cream
- 1/2 cup grated Parmesan cheese
- 2 cups baby spinach leaves
- Fresh parsley, chopped, for garnish (optional)

Instructions:

1. Heat olive oil in a large skillet over medium-high heat.

2. Season the chicken breast pieces with salt and pepper to taste.

3. Add the seasoned chicken breast pieces to the skillet and cook until they are browned on all sides and cooked through, about 5-6 minutes. Remove the chicken from the skillet and set aside.

4. In the same skillet, add minced garlic and cook for about 1 minute until fragrant.

5. Add linguine pasta to the skillet, breaking it in half if needed to fit. Pour chicken broth over the pasta and stir well.

6. Bring the mixture to a boil, then reduce the heat to medium-low. Cover the skillet and let it simmer for about 10-12 minutes, stirring occasionally, until the pasta is cooked al dente and most of the liquid has been absorbed.

7. Stir in heavy cream and grated Parmesan cheese until the sauce is creamy and well combined.

8. Add baby spinach leaves to the skillet and stir until they are wilted.

9. Return the cooked chicken breast pieces to the skillet and stir to combine with the pasta and sauce.

10. Once everything is heated through and well combined, remove the skillet from the heat.

11. Serve the One-Pot Creamy Garlic Chicken Pasta hot, garnished with chopped fresh parsley if desired.

12. Enjoy your delicious and easy single-skillet meal!

98. Stuffed Bell Peppers

Ingredients:
- 4 large bell peppers, any color
- 1 tablespoon olive oil
- 1 onion, diced
- 2 cloves garlic, minced
- 1 lb (450g) ground beef or turkey
- 1 cup cooked rice (white or brown)
- 1 cup diced tomatoes
- 1 cup tomato sauce
- 1 teaspoon dried oregano
- 1 teaspoon dried basil
- Salt and pepper to taste
- 1 cup shredded cheese (such as cheddar or mozzarella)
- Fresh parsley, chopped, for garnish (optional)

Instructions:

1. Preheat your oven to 375°F (190°C).

2. Cut the tops off the bell peppers and remove the seeds and membranes. Set aside.

3. In a large skillet, heat olive oil over medium heat.

4. Add diced onion to the skillet and cook for about 3-4 minutes until softened.

5. Add minced garlic to the skillet and cook for another minute until fragrant.

6. Add ground beef or turkey to the skillet and cook until browned, breaking it up with a spoon as it cooks.

7. Stir in cooked rice, diced tomatoes, tomato sauce, dried oregano, dried basil, salt, and pepper. Cook for another 5 minutes, stirring occasionally, until heated through.

8. Remove the skillet from the heat and spoon the filling into the hollowed-out bell peppers, dividing it evenly among them.

9. Sprinkle shredded cheese over the top of each stuffed bell pepper.

10. Place the stuffed bell peppers upright in the skillet, nestling them close together.

11. Cover the skillet with a lid or aluminum foil and transfer it to the preheated oven.

12. Bake for about 25-30 minutes until the bell peppers are tender and the cheese is melted and bubbly.

13. Once cooked, remove the skillet from the oven.

14. Serve the Stuffed Bell Peppers hot, garnished with chopped fresh parsley if desired. Enjoy your delicious and easy single-skillet Stuffed Bell Peppers!

99. Skillet Ratatouille Quinoa

Ingredients:
- 1 cup quinoa, rinsed
- 2 cups vegetable broth
- 2 tablespoons olive oil
- 1 onion, diced
- 2 cloves garlic, minced
- 1 eggplant, diced
- 1 zucchini, diced
- 1 yellow squash, diced
- 1 bell pepper, diced
- 1 can (14 oz/400g) diced tomatoes
- 2 tablespoons tomato paste
- 1 teaspoon dried thyme
- 1 teaspoon dried oregano
- Salt and pepper to taste
- Fresh basil leaves, chopped, for garnish (optional)

Instructions:

1. In a large skillet, heat olive oil over medium heat.

2. Add diced onion to the skillet and cook for about 3-4 minutes until softened.

3. Add minced garlic to the skillet and cook for another minute until fragrant.

4. Add diced eggplant, zucchini, yellow squash, and bell pepper to the skillet. Cook for about 5-7 minutes until the vegetables are softened.

5. Stir in diced tomatoes, tomato paste, dried thyme, dried oregano, salt, and pepper. Mix well to combine.

6. Add rinsed quinoa to the skillet and stir to combine with the vegetable mixture.

7. Pour vegetable broth over the quinoa and vegetables, ensuring everything is submerged.

8. Bring the mixture to a boil, then reduce the heat to low. Cover the skillet and let it simmer for about 15-20 minutes, or until the quinoa is cooked and the liquid is absorbed.

9. Once cooked, remove the skillet from the heat.

10. Garnish the Skillet Ratatouille Quinoa with chopped fresh basil leaves if desired.

11. Serve hot as a main dish or as a side.

12. Enjoy your delicious and easy single-skillet Skillet Ratatouille Quinoa!

100. Lemon Butter Chicken and Orzo

Ingredients:
- 2 boneless, skinless chicken breasts
- Salt and pepper to taste
- 1 tablespoon olive oil
- 2 cloves garlic, minced
- 1 cup uncooked orzo pasta
- 2 cups chicken broth
- Zest of 1 lemon
- Juice of 1 lemon
- 2 tablespoons unsalted butter
- 1/4 cup grated Parmesan cheese
- Fresh parsley, chopped, for garnish (optional)

Instructions:

1. Season the chicken breasts with salt and pepper to taste.

2. In a large skillet, heat olive oil over medium-high heat.

3. Add the seasoned chicken breasts to the skillet and cook for about 5-6 minutes on each side until they are golden brown and cooked through. Remove the chicken from the skillet and set aside.

4. In the same skillet, add minced garlic and cook for about 1 minute until fragrant.

5. Add uncooked orzo pasta to the skillet and toast it for about 2-3 minutes until lightly golden.

6. Pour chicken broth into the skillet, along with lemon zest and lemon juice. Stir well to combine.

7. Bring the mixture to a simmer, then reduce the heat to low. Cover the skillet and let it cook for about 10-12 minutes, stirring occasionally, until the orzo is cooked and most of the liquid is absorbed.

8. Once the orzo is cooked, stir in unsalted butter and grated Parmesan cheese until melted and well combined.

9. Return the cooked chicken breasts to the skillet and nestle them into the orzo.

10. Cover the skillet and let it simmer for another 2-3 minutes until the chicken is heated through.

11. Once cooked through, remove the skillet from the heat. Garnish the Lemon Butter Chicken and Orzo with chopped fresh parsley if desired.

12. Serve hot, with any remaining lemon butter sauce spooned over the top. Enjoy your delicious and easy single-skillet Lemon Butter Chicken and Orzo!

Thank you